OXFORD MEDIC

Get Slim a

Get Slim and Stay Slim

The Psychology of Weight Control

JENNIFER J. ASHCROFT
Principal Lecturer in Clinical Psychology
Lancashire Polytechnic

and

J. BARRIE ASHCROFT
Head of Psychological Services
Moss Side Hospital, Liverpool

Oxford New York Tokyo
OXFORD UNIVERSITY PRESS
1989

Oxford University Press, Walton Street, Oxford OX2 6DP
Oxford New York Toronto
Delhi Bombay Calcutta Madras Karachi
Petaling Jaya Singapore Hong Kong Tokyo
Nairobi Dar es Salaam Cape Town
Melbourne Auckland
and associated companies in
Berlin Ibadan

Oxford is a trade mark of Oxford University Press

Published in the United States
by Oxford University Press, New York

British Library Cataloguing in Publication Data
Ashcroft, Jennifer J.
Get slim and stay slim: the psychology of weight control.
1. Physical fitness. Slimming. Diet. Psychological aspects
1. Title II. Ashcroft, J. Barrie (James Barrie), 1944–
613.2'5'019
ISBN 0–19–261738–9

Library of Congress Cataloging in Publication Data
(Data available)

Set by Cambrian Typesetters, Frimley, Surrey
Printed in Great Britain by
The Guernsey Press Co. Ltd.,
Guernsey, Channel Islands.

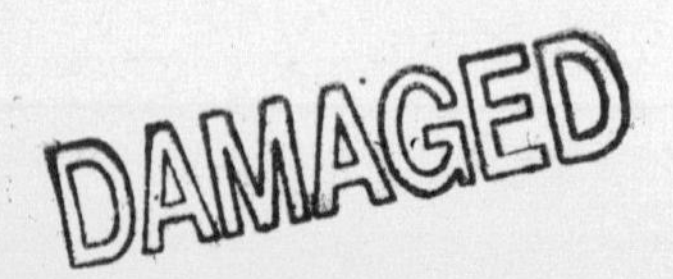

To Caroline, Chloë, and Henry

Preface

Weight control is a major problem for many people. Obesity is a significant health hazard but even mild degrees of overweight can cause great personal distress. Although there are many diets available which can aid weight reduction, they often have disadvantages. First, slimmers have to assess whether or not a diet is nutritionally sound. Assuming it is, the second problem which confronts them is maintaining the diet until all the weight is lost. The third and final obstacle is to keep the fat off once the diet has finished.

This book helps slimmers to overcome all the above problems. It contains a clear description of the most up-to-date research on nutrition and gives the reader an idea of the right kinds of food for maximum health. It also shows how personal food preferences can be incorporated into a good balanced diet. From information given on meal planning, dieters can piece together a diet to suit their own particular food tastes and life-styles. Detailed meal plans are also available for those who would prefer to follow a set diet rather than devise their own programme.

Recent research has shown exercise to be a valuable aid to weight control. Unfortunately, some overweight people find physical exercise aversive. However, there are easy ways of increasing physical activity which speed up weight loss, improve body shape and enhance well-being. Such methods are outlined for slimmers to incorporate into their regime if they wish to use them. All the basic information on the assessment of ideal weight, diet, nutrition, and exercise is described in Part I of this book.

Keeping to a weight-reducing regime is usually difficult. In the past, this issue has largely been avoided; this book is different because it tackles the problem directly. There are psychological methods which are proven to be effective in helping people change behaviour, relearn habits, and actually come to prefer the healthy life-style conducive to maintaining a slim figure. The second part of the book teaches dieters exactly how to establish the self-control necessary to lose weight. Will-power is something that can be enhanced. Slimmers can learn techniques to increase motivation and establish a steady weight loss until the target weight is reached. Such techniques will also ensure that correct weight is maintained once the goal has been achieved.

This book is for anyone who is overweight or anyone who wishes to help an overweight person to lose weight. It does not matter if the weight problem is small or large, if dieting has never been tried before or if a good many diets have been attempted over a period of many years. To stay with a weight reducing regime and be happy with it is a major achievement. It takes skill and determination. This book is different from other diet books because it teaches the psychological skills required for dieting and helps to establish the necessary determination to reach target weight and then enjoy staying there.

Wigan J. J. A.
September 1988 J. B. A.

Contents

Part I

Some basic facts about healthy eating, exercise, and weight control

1

A picture of the problem

Are you happy with yourself, with the way you look? Are you as fit, healthy, and content as you could be? Most people nowadays are aware of some of the basic rules of healthy living. Who has not, at some point, decided to diet, or to change to low-fat, low-sugar food, or to start a new sport or exercise routine? There is plenty on television, in magazines, and in books to encourage you to alter your health-related habits. So why are people still overweight? Why are their eating habits much the same as ever? Why do most adults take insufficient physical exercise? Basically, it is not enough to tell people what good eating entails, and just hope that they will get on with it. Nor is it enough to give them details of exercise and sport and then assume that they will simply become more active. If you are unused to exercise, it hurts. If you love sweet or fatty foods, it is difficult to switch to healthier alternatives. They just do not taste as nice. Losing excess weight entails cutting down on the things you enjoy. So most people break their diets.

But it is possible to change, actually to alter your food preferences, to learn to enjoy exercise, and to achieve an appropriate body weight. Most people fail to change because they know little about how to alter their behaviour. But there is a whole science devoted to the study of behavioural control, and if you can learn something about your own psychology, what motivates you to change, the whole process of becoming healthier, of achieving a new, slim shape, will be very much easier. People's eating habits and food preferences are learned; they are habits that become ingrained over a period of years. However, whatever has been learned can be unlearned. You can then go on to establish new, healthier tastes, better health-promoting habits. Many dieters fail because they try too hard, too quickly. Learning to change the habits of a lifetime will take longer than a week or a month. If you give yourself six months to a year to understand yourself better, gradually to alter your eating and exercise behaviour, you will become slim and healthy and you will stay that way. The whole process will be easy and it will be fun.

Before you can begin the process of change, you need to understand something of your present behaviour, your attitudes towards food and dieting. If you start a diet or an exercise routine, such actions are statements about the way you view yourself. You are to some extent unhappy about your body and your health and you want to improve. This is fine. However, many people who start a health regime stop it before it is due to end. They fail. They break their diet, often with a binge. They feel terrible and so perhaps decide to try twice as hard tomorrow. Tomorrow comes and there is an even stronger pressure to succeed. It is that feeling of pressure and strain, coupled usually with extreme hunger, that makes people break their diets yet again. It is not weight that is lost, but self-esteem. This pattern of behaviour, typical of so many dieters, is not just bad for physical health, it is detrimental to psychological and social well-being too.

Why, then, do people behave this way? The answer is that they are dissatisfied with themselves. They do not want to give up, to throw in the towel, to admit defeat. This is an admirable characteristic. As you are reading this, the chances are that you, too, have tried diets, failed (at least in the long term), and then restarted. Of course, not everyone is so obsessed with body size that they are constantly on the 'yo-yo' of diet, break diet, diet, break diet, and so on. At one extreme is the person who starts a diet every morning and has broken it by the evening. Not quite so bad is the man or woman who starts a diet every Monday, is quite good until Friday, breaks out into wild eating over the weekend, and starts again on Monday. Somewhere further up the scale is the seasonal dieter who goes on a diet in spring to get rid of the Christmas over-indulgence; in summer to get ready for the beach; in autumn to lose the fat gained from too many chips, ice-creams, and Tequila sunrises on holiday; and in early winter to help prepare for the Christmas binge. At the farthest end of the scale is the person who tries to improve his or her shape only once or twice a year, perhaps even less. No matter where on the scale you are, you almost certainly share experiences with the other folk trying to change their shape and their health. Every now and again you feel dissatisfied with the way you look or feel. You diet, or perhaps just try to change to better food, or to increase exercise. You probably do stick to your new regime for a short while. You start to feel benefits. You are a bit trimmer, more agile, better looking. Nevertheless you also feel pressure on you to go back to the old ways. Those pressures come partly from within. You feel hungry; you want to eat more; your muscles ache after exercise, so you miss a few sessions. Pressures also come from outside. You are invited to a party and after a couple of drinks you decide a few crisps or nuts will not hurt. Then you go the whole hog, have whatever else is available, then stop for a fish-and-chip take-away on the way home. You do not even need anything as obvious as a party to start you on this slippery slope. If you are feeling a little hungry, or a little unhappy (perhaps you have not lost as much weight as you thought you should), then you are susceptible. Just seeing an advertisement for cake or chocolates in a magazine or on television will be enough to push you into the kitchen and straight into the biscuit tin. If nothing is readily available you find yourself trying to thaw out the cheesecake from the bottom of the freezer (nobody will miss it, will they?), or working out how long it will take you to get to the shops and back with a bag-full of goodies.

The truth is that most people break their diet not just once, but many times. Dieters keep trying, going back on some diet or other, because they do not want to give up on themselves. After all, good results do occur, even if they are only temporary. However, the great hope all dieters have is that *this* new diet will be the one that will really work. The literature on dieting reinforces this notion by publishing diets that certainly do work and giving case histories of dieters who have succeeded in getting slim using these methods. Photographs are often shown of the slimmer before and after the diet, and indeed, the marvellous effects are there for us all to see. The problem is that dieting on a standard slimming regime is difficult. For every one person who succeeds there are likely to be dozens and dozens who fail. Of course, no one wants to hear about the failures: it is not such interesting reading!

Common sense should tell you that if you are finding it difficult to diet, so must other people. Think of all the diets that have been published in recent years. Some of them are cranky, but many are nutritionally very sound. If they are so good, so readily available, why isn't everybody slim and healthy by now? It is simply because most diets involve immense change in eating habits and usually some degree of hunger; they are too difficult for most people to maintain long enough to become slim. If you have really strong will-power and become slim, reverting back to your old eating habits often puts the weight straight back on again.

Too many diets also have the disadvantage that they are associated with a drop in metabolic rate; that is in effect, the rate at which you burn up food. The more you diet, the less food you will need to maintain you. Therefore when you finish a diet, returning to eating an average amount, the amount you used to eat to maintain a constant weight, will result in you putting on fat. However, it is possible to lose weight and *not* suffer a large drop in metabolic rate. If fat loss is at a relatively slow, steady, controlled pace *and* if moderate exercise is taken, metabolic rate can be kept at a reasonable level; it might even increase, and you will be fitter, too. The methods of weight control we outline in this book will mean that you can eat reasonable, even large amounts of food, and not get fat, once you have achieved your correct weight. Nor will you have to be running marathons or plunging into the swimming pool every day in order to maintain a reasonable level of exercise to speed weight loss and keep metabolic rate high.

Are you addicted to dieting?

Why is it that people continue to follow dieting regimes that do not work? They want to be slim of course, yet after months or years of dieting failure you would think that it was time to stop trying. There is something in this pattern of behaviour that is very reminiscent of some addictive or compulsive behaviours. Let us take gambling as an example. Most compulsive gamblers are not hugely successful. That is, they do not become millionaires and then stop gambling. Many of them are in fact very poor and can ill afford their habit. One school of thought within psychology is that we tend to get hooked into behaviour patterns if they produce intermittent rewards. That is, when success occurs occasionally, not every time, and in a fairly random fashion, the behaviour that has produced this variable success becomes very ingrained and is difficult to eradicate. This certainly seems to be the case with some kinds of gambling. There also seems to be this addictive aspect to some kinds of dieting behaviour. Some diets are easier to stick to than others; some give better results than others. It is fairly unpredictable at the start of any new diet whether this one will give success. Will it give lots of success or just a little? Will you get a big weight loss this week, or will it come next week, or not at all? Some diets are not successful at all but some are, even if only for a short time. The outcome always has some degree of uncertainty associated with it. So you keep trying, and trying, and trying.

If you have been hunting for the perfect diet for a very long time it will be difficult to stop, actually to believe that good weight control can be established without resorting to one special diet that you go on (and then, and this is the snag, come off again). However, you *can* learn to change your

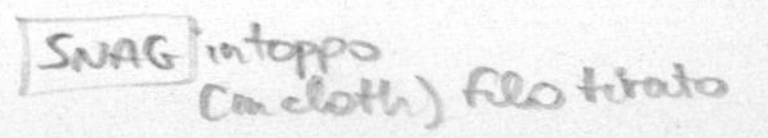

eating behaviour to get slim permanently, to achieve maximum health and good physical shape. But you will achieve success only if you set about it in the right way. There are some very basic psychological principles for you to bear in mind. First, you are likely to succeed in anything only if you make the steps to your goal easy enough to manage. Any new food regime has to be simple to follow if you are to stick with it for any length of time. A diet that involves uncommon foods or drinks, or the same things repeated over and over again, is not a basis for long-term success. Similarly, you will almost certainly break with any regime that results primarily in disagreeable consequences (for example, if you are desperately hungry and thinking about food most of the time). Your new regime should not stop you socializing or from accepting food from others. You should still be able to eat the foods you enjoy. If you are not one for counting calories or fat units, then a diet that involves these things will eventually get broken. You must make your new regime fit in with your current behaviour, your own personal preferences. There is no advantage to making things hard for yourself. This means that if you hate, say, cottage cheese or liver, do not feel that you simply must include these foods in your diet because you have heard that these things are good for you, or because a diet sheet says you must have them. If you do not like a certain food, do not eat it. Simple, you say, yet how many people force down meals on a diet that they would not dream of choosing if they were not on that diet? No wonder diets get broken! The corollary of this is that if you absolutely love certain items like cake or chips, do not ban them from your life for ever, not even for a week. Dieters often feel that high-fat, high-sugar foods are so bad that they should be totally eliminated from a healthy eating plan. However, by being over-zealous with food restriction, the dieter inadvertantly makes a binge on forbidden foods far more likely. You may as well forget the idea of banning things. There is absolutely nothing you cannot eat or drink if you want to. Have what you *like,* and enjoy it without feeling guilty. It is the overall balance of the diet that is important, and a certain quantity of any kind of food or drink can play a part in that balance.

This book is about learning to enjoy eating without feeling guilty, and getting slim and healthy in the process. The odd bar of chocolate is enjoyable for most people and is not going to result in ill health. Of course, some dieters say they cannot help bingeing on such foods. No one doubts that five bars of chocolate eaten for lunch is unhealthy eating. Usually however, most of this type of eating results from over-restriction beforehand, too much hunger, too many favourite foods banned. What does the fifth, or tenth, or fifteenth bar of chocolate in a binge really taste like? Is it slowly savoured and really enjoyed, a splendid taste to satisfy the hunger pangs? Or is it gulped down quickly, before someone comes in and points an accusing finger? This habit of bingeing must be broken. It is a thing that very many dieters do; it is a learnt behaviour resulting primarily from over-restriction of food. You will only be successful with weight control in the long term if you allow yourself to eat foods you enjoy as part of a well-balanced regime. It is also essential never to get so hungry that you lose control.

So, the first psychological principle is to make your goals attainable. In the case of dieting, do not force yourself to diet in a way that involves too much hunger or deprivation. A second principle is that a difficult task (and nobody doubts that dieting can be very difficult) is far easier to accomplish if it is broken down into small, manageable pieces. Unfortunately, most dieters are either off a diet or on it. They swop over from one state (usually over-eating or having lots of high-sugar, high-fat foods) to another, quite separate, diet state (under-eating, with little fat or sugar). Over-eating is considered bad by the dieter, while the slimming regime is difficult but good and virtuous. Everything is seen in black and white. Over-eating involves eating foods you like, convenience foods, take-away dinners, going out to parties or for meals (but you think this is bad and behaving this way makes you feel guilty). On the other hand dieting, which is good, involves you eating foods you do not much like, staying at home, feeling miserable. What a dilemma!

This sad state of affairs does not have to continue. Consider the way you eat, exercise, and socialize when not dieting. Just work on this and forget about the restrictive diet side of the equation. The idea is to emphasize the positive aspects of your present, non-diet, way of eating. It cannot be all bad. After all, you have managed to survive for years without suffering from severe vitamin deficiency—scurvy, rickets, or such things. There is a chapter later on that will help you pinpoint the good aspects of your everyday eating habits. Next, in easy stages, you will need to reshape some of your food preferences. We all learn to like certain tastes, certain textures in the foods we eat. If you carefully plan a new health regime that slowly introduces slight modifications to your usual meals, perhaps to try different ways of cooking food, to have slightly larger portions of vegetables and fruit, you will eventually find that your food preferences change slightly, enough to tip the balance from an unhealthy diet (too high in fat and sugar, too low in fibre), to a healthy one that will help you attain and then maintain a slim figure. It is important to make changes at a pace with which you can easily cope. Where many dieters fall down is that they concentrate on cutting down on food, cutting out pleasure from their lives. Instead, we feel that you should emphasize easy, gradual introduction of steps to enhance your health, to make eating more of a pleasure, and weight control a natural consequence of this new way of life.

A third and important principle is that you should give yourself plenty of reward for your success. The usual reward for keeping to a diet is in-built; you lose weight! Unfortunately the punishment for breaking a diet is also in-built; you put weight back on. Your aim, though, is not simply to lose as much weight as you can in as short a time as possible. You want something better, slightly more complex, and longer-lasting than what the average diet has to offer. You want to enjoy food, not to feel pressured into eating prescribed foods at prescribed times. You want to eat in a way you like. You do not want to be hungry. You want to be slim and you want to stay that way. To achieve all this is going to take time, patience, and careful planning. However, the method we advocate, that helps you achieve all your aims, is itself enjoyable. The process of gaining control over your health-related habits should be easy and fun. You can reward yourself with little prizes on the way to your ultimate goal. The process of trying new ways of eating, new recipes, still enjoying your favourite foods, and feeling more trim and healthy every day, should also be a reward in itself.

If you have never dieted before and want to lose weight

It is just possible that you are one of those rare people who has never seriously tried to diet. Now this is a little unlikely. With women especially, there is a great deal of social pressure to conform to a certain physical shape. Girls in their early teens or even younger often try to lose weight. Dieting almost seems an integral part of adult female behaviour. Even if they have not gone through this early stage of becoming interested in dieting, women often find that after the birth of a baby they have a little excess fat to lose and this often marks the beginning of an obsession with shape and with dieting. Men and women both tend to put on weight in middle-age, when exercise becomes less frequent. However, gaining weight is not an inevitable part of getting older.

If you have never dieted before, or have had just one or two unsuccessful attempts, please do not start on the 'yo-yo' of losing weight, gaining weight, losing weight that we described earlier. Now is the ideal time to review your total eating behaviour and your exercise habits. You can then plan the small, easy, enjoyable steps back to good physical shape.

Why bother making changes?

Some people give up dieting completely. Who can blame them when most traditional methods of weight control fail in the long term? Others, seeing what so many people put themselves through in the quest for slimness, just decide not to bother. Clearly too many diets involve deprivation that is so severe that the dieter breaks away from them.

Other people, who are perhaps close to, or even at the right weight, are still not necessarily eating well. We are all bombarded through the media about the nutritional adequacy of the food we eat. Certainly, there is very good evidence that we eat too much sugar, too much saturated fat, too much salt, and not enough fibre. Our appallingly high rate of circulatory disorders (including stroke and heart attack) is linked to an over-rich diet and relative lack of exercise. Even children suffer because of the inadequacy of the food they eat. Their teeth suffer decay; disease of the arteries can start in childhood; even hyperactive behaviour may be partially linked to diet.

Despite these problems most people get by and have a life expectancy of about 70 to 80 years. Isn't this enough? Actually it is wrong to think that your present diet will necessarily lead to a long and productive life. People (women as well as men) often have fatal heart attacks at an earlier age. A stroke does not come suddenly at the age of 75 or 80 and finish life. It can come much earlier and lead to physical and mental disability. Who wants to spend the last 10 or 20 years of their existence incontinent, or unable to speak properly, or with severe memory problems, or unable to walk?

Strokes and heart attacks are not the only problems. For example, diseases such as diabetes, rheumatism, and arthritis all have links with diet. Being over-weight, and eating and exercising inappropriately, will make many diseases worse and will affect the quality of life. So it is worth making changes, but it is essential that in the process you do not make your everyday life a misery. You sometimes hear people say that it is not worth eating differently, or getting to the right weight; they say they prefer a short and happy life to a long and miserable one. This argument might have something in it if the road to fitness were hard and difficult to achieve. However, if you set about it in the right way it can be an easy road, a pleasant country ramble rather than an attempt to scale Everest. A change to a healthier style of living can be simple to achieve and can be enjoyable too. Follow the advice we give in this book and you will attain all your health and fitness goals.

2

So you want to change

The first thing to do is to form a realistic picture of how you want your physical shape to change. There is more to looking better than losing weight. Think about how people look after a period of sickness and diarrhoea. They go pale with shrunken eyes; they look ill rather than slimmer. Good weight control *must* be coupled with good nutrition and adequate exercise to maintain muscle tone. Eat well and your complexion will become clear and radiant, your eyes will sparkle, your whole appearance will improve. You might also like to consider your overall image. If your face changes shape, perhaps a different hair style would suit you better. If you wear spectacles, how about some new frames or tinted lenses? Have you considered contact lenses? Presumably your clothes will need to be altered or some new ones purchased. Should you change your style of dress? Most overweight people chose to hide their size with baggy tops and loose, stretchy slacks, long skirts, or tent-shaped dresses. Learning which fashions will suit the new you is bound to take time. Fortunately you have that time. As you slowly lose weight you can programme little rewards for yourself, like a visit to the hairdresser for a restyle, new make-up, new glasses, a tour of the clothes shops to try out new styles, and so on.

As you start to succeed in changing your shape, you will find your self-esteem and general enjoyment of life grows. Your personal relationships should improve. You should feel capable of doing more and therefore you will become more of a busy, dynamic person. You might like to consider how these personal qualities are developing as a side-effect to your health programme. Expect that generally things will change for the better.

However, try not to expect unrealistic changes. If you are a fifty-year old person, losing some weight and doing more exercise will improve your looks and your outlook on life, but you will not look twenty years old. If you have problems socializing, looking better might give you more confidence but you still might have to give yourself that final push to get out there and start mingling. If you are in your late teens or are doing a further education course and you are extremely worried about examinations, you are going to have to find a way to tackle academic stress that does not involve eating and drinking too much. In fact, people often cope with any stress by turning to food or drink for comfort. It would be much better to learn other coping methods. You can learn how to be a better decision-maker, how to plan and organize things efficiently, how to relax, how to take your mind off your problems by engrossing yourself in other things. Developing such skills will stand you in good stead for when some stressful situation occurs to which you would normally respond by eating a box of chocolates or downing four or five gin and tonics or glasses of beer.

What overweight people think slim people are like

The obese, even the mildly chubby, sometimes regard slim people as veritable paragons of virtue when it comes to food. The myth goes that the slim person likes, indeed prefers, foods like cottage cheese, plain yogurt, salads, crispbreads, low-fat spreads, and other foods so often described in diets. In fact (the myth persists), even if the slim person does not especially like these foods, he or she sticks with them for a large part of the time in order to maintain a trim figure.

The average over-weight person tends to imagine the slim person's day to go something like this. Ms or Mr Trim wakes up for an early morning drink, has tea or coffee with either no milk or skimmed milk and definitely no sugar. Breakfast is something that sounds healthy such as a wholewheat cereal with no sugar added, or a thin slice of unbuttered toast with a free-range egg on top. After this virtuous start Ms or Mr Trim never, of course, succumbs to a biscuit or cake half-way through the morning. Lunch will be fairly small and might feature a salad or small sandwich with a low-fat filling, or yogurt and fruit. Not many people make it through to the evening meal without any snack, so, being realistic, the overweight person imagines Ms or Mr Trim indulges in a light, healthy snack such as fresh fruit in the afternoon; certainly not a bar of chocolate. The final meal of the day is usually the largest for most people. However, it is still difficult to imagine the slim person going for for a real blow-out, or having dinner, going to the pub, then calling into an Indian Restaurant for a further meal before going home. It is far easier to imagine Ms or Mr Trim tucking into a low-fat meal, perhaps featuring fish or chicken accompanied by vegetables. Dessert, when it is taken, might be fruit or yogurt rather than, say, treacle pudding or Black Forest Gateaux.

Now it is not always possible to be so absolutely in control of food intake that the slim person can guarantee each meal will be a low fat, low sugar, and fairly low-calorie affair. So the myth has it that Ms or Mr Trim very carefully calculates how much food (or how many calories) to forgo in order to afford an occasional large meal (on holiday or at Christmas for example). And, if by some misfortune, he or she miscalculates and dares to put on even a tiny amount of excess fat, this is immediately dieted off within a week of it first appearing.

What a wonderful person Ms or Mr Trim appears to be! Certainly, you do read the odd story that describes a person behaving in just the way we have outlined. Some people manage to live in this virtuous way for a short time; the very rare person for years. However, we cannot stress enough how unusual it is to find anyone who conforms to the stereotyped Ms or Mr Trim image. Most slim people do not behave this way. It is almost impossible to keep such a tight regime going for any length of time. Most people, even slim people, over-indulge from time to time. Where a person does become so obsessional that this never happens, there is often some other problem. That is, it is sometimes found that when there is a part of a person's life which is difficult or impossible to control, he or she will channel the need to exercise control onto some other aspect of behaviour such as food intake. So, are we saying that it is somehow abnormal or freakish to be able to stick to a healthy regime and remain slim? No, we are not! Some rare people remain slim by staying with a very restrictive way of eating. However, by far the majority of slim people eat in a relatively relaxed, rather haphazard style that is not governed by special rules. They snack between meals. They eat chocolate, cake, and sweets. They fry food. They sometimes eat too much. Therefore let us consider next not the myth, but the reality of the eating habits of slim people.

What slim people are actually like in terms of food intake

Food preferences are obviously a very individual matter. However, some foods are pretty universally popular. Most of us like sweet foods like confectionery. Fatty foods, like rich sauces, many types of meat, and cheese, are also popular. Some products, such as cake, chocolate, and biscuits, are sources of high levels of both fat and sugar.

At a general evolutionary level it is quite adaptive for a species to seek out foods that provide reasonable amounts of nutrients and give high energy levels. Food should supply a relatively high number of calories to match our high energy requirements. Unlike some animals, such as cows or sheep, that spend hours and hours chewing low-energy food such as grass in order to acquire adequate nutrition, we can consume enough high-calorie food in a relatively small period of time to supply our daily requirements, thus freeing us to do other things with our day besides eat.

Fairly basic foods like meat, fish, eggs, milk, vegetables, fruit, rice, bread, and pasta provide reasonable amounts of nutrients and have appropriate calorie content for our needs. Problems arise, however, when our modern society tries to make food even more palatable by making it fattier or sweeter than it should be. Foods rich in fat or refined sugar might seem very attractive but usually prove to be far too tempting for our own good; it is far too easy to over-indulge in these kinds of food. Slim people, like those who are overweight, are lured by modern food products. They add sugar to their breakfast cereal (or buy a variety which is sugar-coated). The milk added to the cereal is probably ordinary full-fat silver top milk. The lunch-time meal will probably be fairly high in fat (such as a pasty or pie; or cheese sandwiches with a generous spread of butter or margarine on the bread; or fish and chips). Afternoon snacks might include a biscuit or a piece of cake. The evening meal is also fairly high in fat and sugar. It might include chips or other food fried in fat. The main meal is often followed by something sweet.

Slim people generally eat the same kinds of food that fatter people like to eat. The difference between the two groups is that slim individuals tend to get the overall balance between food intake and energy expenditure right, while overweight people generally do not. The slim person will have a couple of chocolates in the day, then stop. Why not save some for tomorrow? The fatter person is more likely to eat a larger number, and will continue eating after hunger is satisfied. If the diet is broken why not make the most of it before the diet begins again tomorrow? The slim person, if busy, might delay or even miss a meal. The dieter has learned to be more obsessed by food and would not omit a meal. If the slim person has eaten a really large meal, he or she will naturally be very full and will perhaps not eat again until hunger really returns; in addition this type of person might take a little exercise to 'work off' the food. The overweight person, on the other hand, is usually not so mindful of internal sensations as a cue for eating or abstaining, and is less likely to take exercise as an antidote to excess indulgence.

Slim people generally eat according to appetite, in a fairly relaxed fashion not governed by rules or diet sheets. They eat reasonably generous meals and they snack in between. However, because they are cued by internal sensations of hunger and satiation, and they respond reasonably well to those cues, they are not likely to overeat. Also, eating is not likely to be viewed as a cardinal sin. The occasional over-indulgence will not make the person guilt-ridden. Their attitude to food tends to be fairly relaxed.

Contrary to popular opinion the slim person's weight is not exactly the same each day, totally stable. Occasionally a little extra body fat is added. However, the human body can take minor fluctuations in weight with no ill effect. Occasionally we all suffer from influenza or a bout of sickness, which naturally results in a drop in weight. The tiny gains in weight should ideally be balanced out by these losses. The amounts of fat-gain and fat-loss involved are usually too small to show. Overweight individuals tend not to be so relaxed about fluctuations in body size as slim people.

How to be healthier

Is the goal of an overweight person to be like the picture of a slim person such as we have just described? In terms of having a relaxed attitude to food the answer is yes. In terms of learning to eat (and to stop eating!) by listening to the body's demands and signals, the answer is yes. In terms of learning to enjoy food, and not feel guilty about eating, the answer is also yes. However, recent research indicates that the slim person is not necessarily eating in a way to promote maximum health. Because of modern methods of food preparation and presentation, and the trend to make foods more appealing by adding saturated fat and refined sugar, slim people as well as their weightier friends are likely to be eating too rich a diet. Those people who do manage to stay slim but who are eating average foods, highly processed, high in fat, sugar, and salt but low in fibre, are likely to be damaging their health in the long term.

Any high-fat, high-sugar way of eating is likely to be providing fewer nutrients than a low-fat, low-sugar regime with similar overall calorie content. (Sugar in particular provides 'empty calories', that is, it provides energy unaccompanied by protein, minerals, or vitamins.) Malnutrition need not manifest itself in the short term as severe disease. Low-grade malnutrition (slightly fewer vitamins and minerals than you need; too much fat and sugar and too little fibre) can show itself in small, insidious ways. You might feel below par, that 'washed-out' feeling; your resistance to infection could well be affected; you will not have the zest for life that you should have.

The aim of everyone, irrespective of weight, should be to modify their eating very slightly to maximize health benefits. These modifications need not be huge. As we said earlier, you can keep on with your favourite foods and you need not formulate strict rules that ban your preferred treats from your life. Once you start eating in a healthier way, good weight control should become much easier.

The meaning of control

There is a commonly held fallacy that taking control of your life in any way, be it in terms of changed food intake, exercise, or anything else, means that you have to be extra-strict and rigid in your approach. Many dieters believe this myth. Hence, if a diet involves calorie restriction to 1000 calories per day, then not 980, not 1020, but exactly the 1000 calories should pass the lips. Foods are meticulously weighed and measured. If it is not calories, it may be fat units or fibre units that are counted, or very exact portions of food.

With rules generally being so rigid it is hardly surprising that diets, and the good intentions that go with them, quickly get left behind. However, taking control does not mean you have to be rigid in your approach to your health. Real control includes flexibility. You need to adapt to the demands of your own particular life-style. If you are under pressure to eat out socially you should be able to do this and include it as part of your regime without having to compensate by going hungry at some time prior to the meal out. If you do not have time to prepare breakfast it should not matter. You can omit breakfast if that is your personal preference and still be healthy. If you are out shopping, get tired, and are tempted by a cake and a cup of coffee, your overall health regime should not suffer because you decide to enjoy yourself in this way occasionally. If you are given a box of chocolates they should not represent ruin and damnation. Enjoy them as a part of your total balanced diet. If, when you come home from work or a hard afternoon outdoors, and you want to prepare a healthy, appetizing meal in ten minutes flat, you should be able to do so. Healthy meals can be as quick and easy to prepare as their less nutritious counterparts. Only when your approach to good health can be adapted to all your own requirements (and your family's requirements too if this is relevant), will you really succeed in attaining your goals.

This idea of flexibility applies as much to exercise as it does to food. Any rigid scheme that means exact amounts of specific exercise must be carried out each day is usually doomed to failure. What if one day you just do not have time? Or you catch a cold and you just do not feel up to it? Your beautiful scheme is ruined. You let things lapse for a few days more. You lose motivation. Before you know it you are back where you started, in the armchair in front of the television consuming a large box of your favourite chocolate assortment as a comfort for your injured self-esteem. Real control of exercise, like real control of food intake, needs to be flexible enough to take into account the unpredictability of life, your fluctuations in mood, the vagaries of fortune.

The evolution of a new life-style

Weight change

Any changes you make to your health-related habits should be relatively easy to achieve. All the small modifications should add up over a period of time to make major achievements.

If you are trying to alter the habits of a lifetime, expect the process to be slow. If you have had a weight problem for a long time, do not expect a miracle in a few weeks. Let us take an example of someone who is now thirty-five years old and who has been somewhat overweight, say between 15 and 30 lb, for at least ten years. Any diet that takes this weight off in a month or two will probably not be successful in the long term. Unless the dieter permanently modifies his or her eating behaviour, any weight lost is likely to be regained. However, if he or she decides to evolve a new style of weight control, and aims for a slow and steady loss, the weight is more likely to stay off. Crash diets are very difficult to keep to for any length of time. You need to find a food regime that is so easy and pleasurable that you can keep to it indefinitely. Remember, a loss of between 2 and 4 lb per month adds up to a 24–48 lb drop in a year, 48–96 lb over two years. This should solve most weight problems! This cure is one that will last; you need never diet again.

Food change

As well as losing weight, you will also be changing to a better quality diet and monitoring food intake. This does not mean writing down everything you eat. We shall show you later how to choose suitable goals. Changes should always be small, easy, and enjoyable. For example, rather than concentrate on food restriction, you might choose to concentrate primarily on increasing consumption of filling, high-fibre, low-fat foods like wholemeal bread or jacket potatoes. Such foods do not deserve the bad reputation they have gained over the years; eating them more often might well serve to curb the appetite for fatty foods or confectionery.

Another helpful approach is to substitute some low-fat foods for their high-fat counterparts, for example, have semi-skimmed or skimmed milk instead of full-fat milk.

Here again, you might start by changing the proportions of various foods in meals. For example, if one evening you had planned a three-egg omelette filled with cheese and accompanied by peas or baked beans, why not use only two eggs, half the quantity of cheese, but more peas or beans; you could add a slice of wholemeal bread too. This way you increase the variety in your diet, increase fibre (with the extra pulses and bread) and decrease saturated fat (present in eggs and cheese). With a little knowledge you can make very healthy changes to your diet without having to alter radically your whole way of eating. The many routes to a healthier diet will be described later in the book. You can then choose whichever routes you think will be best suited to your own particular life-style. Should you cook for others beside yourself, they too will benefit from the new food regime.

Exercise change

If you are going to improve your fitness you will almost certainly need to increase your exercise level. However, if you hate exercise, be assured that the whole enterprise is not necessarily doomed to failure. As you eat better and become slimmer you will automatically find activity more enjoyable. Almost without thinking about it you will be doing more moving around, walking faster, taking stairs without strain, and so on. If, on top of this, you can find an additional sport or exercise you enjoy, so much the better. Something as small as a brisk fifteen-minute walk each day can make a big difference to health.

From now on, the pressure to instigate fast, hard-to-achieve changes is off. No more rigid, over-restrictive diets that leave you hungry and miserable. No excessive exercise regimes that leave you an aching wreck. Instead you can approach better health in an easy, relaxed manner. You must be flexible and open to the suggestions we make. You can expect a few difficulties and the occasional setback. Undoubtedly these will occur. You might try a new recipe and find it awful. A month might go by in which you do not lose as much weight as you had hoped. However, if you keep trying with the plan we outline, you will certainly succeed. You will be able to enjoy the process of acquiring control over your eating and exercise behaviour and the success you gain by losing weight will be long-lasting.

3

Your aim for weight

It is surprisingly difficult to decide on an ideal goal weight for any individual. There are charts and general guides available to help you decide but it is still difficult to pinpoint an exact weight at which you will be just right. However, if you look at all of the various ways of assessing correct body weight, you should develop an idea of a suitable goal weight for you. More importantly, by the time you finish this chapter, you should have a good idea of the right size and shape for your body. Weight is not everything. Someone weighing 9 st (57.2 kg) can have a large proportion of flabby fat or can be trim and taut. It is essential to keep in mind the kind of healthy look you are aiming for, as well as your goal for weight. You must never diet so quickly that you lose the muscle tissue that gives your body its shape, firmness, and definition. There is not much point in weighing less but looking as if you are suffering from some wasting disease. Aim for a healthy diet, an increase in exercise, and slow, steady weight loss to a goal weight and goal shape.

Frame size and ideal weight charts

In order to use weight charts properly you generally need to know your height and also your frame size. Height should not present a problem, but frame size can be difficult to assess. There are various ways of attempting this. The first one is to take the measurement around your wrist as a guide. If you have a small wrist (less than 5.5 in., 14 cm), you have a small frame. If your wrist is between 5.5 in. (14 cm) and 6.5 in. (16 cm) you are medium-framed. Anything over 6.5 in. (16 cm) indicates a large frame. What could be simpler?

However, although this is a quick, easy guide, it is not infallible. For example, small wrists often indicate a small frame, but not always. It might simply be that you are a person with small wrists but a large body frame, wide shoulders, wide rib-cage, and so on. Of course, you might have very large wrists because you are extremely overweight; the measurement may indicate thickness of fat rather than bone size.

Another indicator is the size of your feet. For your height, do you have large, medium, or small feet? Again, this is a very rough estimate, because it might just be, for example, that you have a narrow, small frame, but very large feet underneath it all!

There is yet another, rather unorthodox method of assessing frame size that is much favoured by the overweight. You take an 'Ideal Height' chart and find your height on it. For example, if you are a woman of 5 ft 5 in. (1.65 m) and you weigh 9 st 11 lb (62.1 kg), the chart says you are just right *provided* you have a large frame. If however, you are small-framed, you should be around 8 st 2 lb. (51.7 kg.). And if you are medium-framed you should be 8 st 13 lb. (56.7 kg.). From all the available data in the charts you decide you must be large-framed *because* you weigh 9 st 11 lb. (62.1 kg.). Now, this just might be true for a small minority of women of 5 ft 5 in. (1.65 m) and 9 st 11 lb. (62.1 kg.). However, the probabilities are that you are fooling yourself. You are 5 ft 5 in. (1.65 m), you are 9 st 11 lb. (62.1 kg.), and you are too fat! Probabilities being what they are, you are most likely to be right in assessing frame size if you assume that you are medium-framed. So a woman of 5 ft 5 in. (1.65 m) should probably be somewhere around 8 st 13 lb. (56.7 kg.)

We include here an ideal weight chart (Table 1) to help you assess your own personal goal, but *do remember* that this is a rough estimate only. For the woman in our example, it might just be that in fact she has a very small frame and she should therefore be 8 st 2 lb. (51.7 kg.). Obviously the goal of 8 st 13 lb. (56.7 kg.) would leave her a full 11 lb. (5 kg.) overweight. Charts, then, are only a rough guide to ideal weight. What they definitely *do* indicate are the extremes of weight problems; where your weight falls higher than the amount given under the large-frame weight for your height, or lower than that given for the small-frame weight for your height, then you have problems.

A final, arithmetical method used to estimate correct weight is this. First, work out your weight in kg (multiply your weight in pounds by 0.45 to get this figure). Second,

Table 1 A guide to ideal weight

Women

Height*		Weight†					
		Small frame		Medium frame		Large frame	
ft in		st lb	(kg)	st lb	(kg)	st lb	(kg)
4 9	(1.45)	6 7	(41.3)	7 3	(45.8)	7 11	(49.4)
4 10	(1.47)	6 9	(42.2)	7 5	(46.7)	8 0	(50.8)
4 11	(1.50)	6 11	(43.1)	7 7	(47.6)	8 4	(52.6)
5 0	(1.52)	6 13	(44.0)	7 10	(49.0)	8 7	(54.0)
5 1	(1.55)	7 2	(45.4)	7 13	(50.3)	8 10	(55.3)
5 2	(1.57)	7 5	(46.7)	8 2	(51.7)	8 13	(56.7)
5 3	(1.60)	7 8	(48.1)	8 5	(53.1)	9 3	(58.5)
5 4	(1.63)	7 12	(49.9)	8 9	(54.9)	9 7	(60.3)
5 5	(1.65)	8 2	(51.7)	8 13	(56.7)	9 11	(62.1)
5 6	(1.68)	8 5	(53.1)	9 3	(58.5)	10 2	(64.4)
5 7	(1.70)	8 8	(54.4)	9 7	(60.3)	10 6	(66.2)
5 8	(1.73)	8 12	(56.2)	9 11	(62.1)	10 10	(68.0)
5 9	(1.75)	9 2	(58.1)	10 1	(64.0)	11 11	(70.3)
5 10	(1.78)	9 6	(59.9)	10 5	(65.8)	11 5	(72.2)
5 11	(1.80)	9 9	(61.2)	10 9	(67.6)	11 9	(73.9)
6 0	(1.83)	9 13	(63.0)	10 13	(69.4)	11 13	(75.8)

* Height is measured without shoes
† Weight is measured without clothes

Table 1 (*continued*)

Men

Height* ft in		Weight† Small frame st lb	(kg)	Medium frame st lb	(kg)	Large frame st lb	(kg)
5 1	(1.55)	6 9	(48.5)	8 6	(53.5)	9 3	(58.5)
5 2	(1.57)	7 12	(49.9)	8 9	(54.9)	9 7	(60.3)
5 3	(1.60)	8 1	(51.3)	8 13	(56.7)	9 11	(62.1)
5 4	(1.63)	8 3	(52.2)	9 2	(58.1)	10 1	(64.0)
5 5	(1.65)	8 7	(54.0)	9 6	(59.9)	10 4	(65.3)
5 6	(1.68)	8 10	(55.3)	9 10	(61.7)	10 9	(67.6)
5 7	(1.70)	9 0	(57.2)	10 0	(63.5)	11 0	(69.9)
5 8	(1.73)	9 4	(59.0)	10 4	(65.3)	11 4	(71.7)
5 9	(1.75)	9 8	(60.8)	10 8	(67.1)	11 9	(73.9)
5 10	(1.78)	9 12	(62.6)	10 13	(69.4)	12 0	(76.2)
5 11	(1.80)	10 2	(64.4)	11 3	(71.2)	12 4	(78.0)
6 0	(1.83)	10 6	(66.2)	11 8	(73.5)	12 9	(80.1)
6 1	(1.85)	10 10	(68.0)	11 12	(75.3)	13 0	(82.6)
6 2	(1.88)	11 1	(70.3)	12 3	(77.6)	13 6	(85.3)
6 3	(1.90)	11 6	(72.6)	12 8	(79.8)	14 1	(89.4)
6 4	(1.93)	11 12	(75.3)	13 0	(82.6)	14 7	(92.1)

* Height is measured without shoes
† Weight is measured without clothes

make a note of your height in metres (equivalent to your height in inches multiplied by 0.0254). Next, divide the weight number by the height number. Finally, divide your answer by the height number once again. For women if this final answer is between 19.1 and 20.6 this indicates correct weight for a small frame. If the number is between 20.1 and 22.5, this is fine for a medium frame. With a large frame the final answer should be between 21.4 and 24.6 to indicate correct weight. For men, the numbers are very similar: a small-framed man should be between 19.7 and 21.2; a medium-framed man between 20.7 and 22.9; and a large-framed man between 22.1 and 24.9. If the number you computed for yourself is higher than the top number for your frame size you are overweight.

Here is an example. A woman of 65 inches weighs 132 lb. and thinks she is medium-framed.

Step 1: weight in kg is 132 × 0.45 = 59.4 kg.

Step 2: height in metres is 65 × 0.0254 = 1.65 m.

Step 3: weight divided by height is 5.94/1.65 = 36.

Step 4: the answer from Step 3 divided by the height number again is 36/1.65 = 21.8.

This answer falls within the acceptable range and so indicates that this person is at or reasonably close to her ideal weight.

The problem with all these apparently objective methods of assessing ideal weight is that there is such a wide range of acceptable weights for any given height. These methods, therefore, are only a beginning to your deciding on the right goal weight for you.

What shape are you in right now?

One aid to setting your goal for weight is to assess, as objectively as you can, your present size and appearance. You will have your own body image fixed in your mind. You might view yourself as pretty acceptable, or slightly away from your goal weight, or even as really fat. It is surprisingly rare to find that your body image (that is, how you see yourself in your mind's eye) is a true appraisal of your actual size. You often find, for example, that teenage girls who are just slightly overweight see themselves as massively obese. Even females suffering from anorexia nervosa tend to view their thin, frail bodies as fat and unsightly. Conversely, some people who are a great deal heavier than they should be can persuade themselves that they are just right (or simply 'big framed').

It can be an illuminating experience to find how your mental image of your size differs from the reality. Here are some ways of doing just that.

Measuring body parts

First, write on a piece of paper how you view yourself. If you know your height and weight, write this at the top. Then, *guess* the following statistics: chest (around the fullest part); for women, just under the bust (where the edge of your bra would go); waist (*not* pulling your tummy in as hard as you can); hips; around one thigh, at the widest part at the top; mid-thigh; just above the knee; just below the knee; mid-calf; ankle; the top of one arm (around the widest part); around the arm mid-way between elbow and wrist. When you have guessed all these, get a tape measure and find the real sizes. How many were correct? How many were way out? Of course, it can be difficult to estimate size of, say, an ankle or a calf if you have never done this before. And, having measured, you still will not know if this is average or not. The next step, then, is to ask a good friend (preferably one whose height is about the same as yours and whose appearance you admire) to take his or her own measurements. You can then compare your friend's 'ideal' measurements with your own record.

Assessing the amount of body fat

There are now instruments available to measure body fat. Basically, they are glorified 'pincers', which pinch the skin and find how thick the fat layer is at various points around the body. However, you do not need to invest in expensive gadgets in order to find if you are fat around the middle: sit down on a seat, relax, do not pull your tummy in, and pinch the fat just above your waist. More than an inch or so

(2.5 cm) indicates excess fat. Does your abdomen bulge forward in a little pot shape? Are your thighs dimpled or overlapping the chair seat? Are your knees chubby, with little fatty pads around the top of each knee? Put your arm out straight in front of you. Are there fatty flaps ('bat wings') hanging down from your upper arm? Do you have a fat face? Do you have a double chin? If you are finding that you are answering 'yes' to most of these questions, it is time you took action!

The mirror test

Many people with weight problems avoid full-length mirrors as much as possible. This is a pity because one of the best ways to gauge body size is to stand naked in front of one and take a realistic look at yourself. Get a long mirror fixed to your bathroom or bedroom wall and take a good look at yourself front way on. Do not stand slightly sideways in order to minimize your size. What do you really look like? Next, turn sideways to the mirror. Relax and do not attempt to pull your tummy in hard. Stand as you normally would. Next, use a hand mirror in conjunction with the wall mirror to get a back view of yourself. So, what do you think? Is there room for improvement? This simple appraisal of size is likely to give you a good, accurate picture of physical shape; use it in conjunction with the other methods in this chapter.

Photographs

Do you hate having your photograph taken? Some individuals are not at all photogenic and really do look much better in real life than in pictures. However, there is also the possibility that you do not like looking at your photo because it reminds you of a weight problem that you do not want to face. However, now is the time to face it because you are about to change, to actually help yourself to a better figure. If possible have a friend or your spouse take some photographs. Have at least six done, and wear clothes that do not hide your shape. For women, tight trousers and top or a leotard or swimsuit; for men, swimming trunks would be ideal. Stand the way you usually do. Have the photos taken with the back view, front view and side view. Have some taken sitting down as well. If you do not feel you want to do this it is a great pity but at least do not avoid having your photograph taken as part of the normal course of events (at weddings, parties, social events). Knowing how the camera portrays you will give you a better idea of how others see you.

Setting goals

By now you should have a clearer picture of your current size and shape. Write down specific goals in a notebook or diary. These goals will be for weight and also possibly for size, i.e. your 'vital statistics'. Even if you are more or less an appropriate weight to begin with, you can benefit from exercise to tone the muscles. You might like to stay the same weight but change your shape. You could exercise to increase the amount of lean muscle tissue and decrease the amount of fat in your body. This will also have the effect of increasing your metabolic rate; in effect you will be able to eat much more yet not become fat. Obviously there are limits to what you can achieve, but you will not know what those limits are until you embark upon a programme of good nutritious eating and appropriate exercise. Suffice it to say that there are very few people who are at present at their full potential for good health and good looks. You do not know what you can achieve until you try.

Monitoring progress

The easiest way to monitor change is by weighing regularly. However, weight is not the be-all and end-all and you must keep a check on your general shape and fitness. Lose weight too quickly and you will lose muscle tissue as well as fat. You will be physically smaller and able to fit into smaller clothes but you will still be flabby and unfit, or, if you overdo it, you will be little more than skin and bone. Also, at the end of it all you will have to eat like a bird in order to avoid putting back all the fat you lost. So there are many reasons to avoid crash dieting.

Occasionally you may need to revise your goals. As you approach your goal weight you may realize that your original aims were slightly unrealistic. Goals for body size may need minor re-adjustment too. Be as realistic and objective as you can.

Listening to what others say

As your health regime progresses people will start to recognize a change in your shape. You will obviously elicit comments. These will probably be quite variable. They should mostly be complimentary, of course, but you might get the odd envious remark directed your way. If your spouse starts to feel slightly insecure (because other people find you attractive now) he or she might well say you looked better when you were 'cuddly'. Some overweight friends might feel that your success highlights their own failure to slim, so they might try to sabotage your progress.

Generally, if most remarks are positive and you feel you are doing well then you can ignore any negative comments and carry on. However, if virtually everybody (friends and family) start to remark that you are losing too much weight, consider that they might just be right. Reassess your progress and try to make sure your mental body image fits the reality. Attaining maximum health involves much more than aiming for a low weight.

4

Your aim for diet

The first thing most people do when they diet is to cut out many of the foods they like. They concentrate mostly on self-denial, with no cakes, sweets, bread, chocolate, sugar, potatoes, crisps, and so on. The result of this may be that the foods they do choose to eat are very limited. For example, there is the hard-boiled egg diet where four to six eggs are eaten each day. Then there is the grapefruit diet where grapefruit is eaten before each meal. Another variation on repetitious dieting involves having a liquid protein drink instead of a meal. Such diets totally change the person's style of eating. This is unfortunate because what is really wanted is a modification of standard everyday food, leading to a healthier type of eating that can be incorporated permanently into the person's life.

Diets often fail in the long term because they are too demanding on will-power. In some cases they are also nutritionally unsound. And most diets are not flexible enough for you to indulge yourself occasionally.

Rather than concentrate on restrictions it is much easier, at least initially, to consider the positive aspect of healthy eating. Are you having enough fruit, vegetables, low-fat milk, wholegrain bread, and cereals? Does your food supply you with enough calcium, iron, and vitamins? Are you having the right kinds of fats (polyunsatured rather than hard, saturated fats)? It is not enough to rely on vitamin pills and hope for the best. A multi-vitamin and mineral tablet will not be enough to turn an unhealthy diet into a good one. You need to learn some basic facts about nutrition and the balance of different nutrients that you need at meals. Once you start making the slight adjustment necessary to make your normal way of eating healthier, you will automatically be on your way to weight control. Good food control contributes a great deal to good weight control.

The positive aspects of a healthy diet: plenty of the right kinds of food

Protein from animal and plant sources

Virtually everyone has heard about the importance of adequate protein in the diet. Protein is essential for the growth of body cells and for their repair, and for their eventual replacement with new cells. Protein is so important that nearly all diets, no matter what other failings they may have, emphasize adequate protein intake. Most people know the main animal sources of protein and can reel off a basic list: meat, fish, eggs, and dairy products such as milk, yogurt, and cheese. Indeed, until relatively recently a healthy food intake was described as one that included quite heavy protein intake. However, eating large amounts of protein food like red meat, milk, cheese, and eggs also produces a high proportion of saturated fat in the diet, because all these foods are high in saturated fat as well as protein.

So while animal sources of protein are very important, you should try to eat more animal proteins that are low in saturated fat, such as poultry, fish, and low-fat dairy products such as skimmed or semi-skimmed milk and yogurt. Eggs and *lean* red meat are quite acceptable *in moderation*.

Although the diet literature often gives information about animal sources of protein, there is surprisingly little about plant sources. In fact, it is possible to obtain more than enough protein to meet requirements without using animal sources at all. Protein is made up of amino acids; these are the basic units or 'building bricks' for the body to use for cell growth and repair. These bricks are not all the same kind. They come in different types and you need an assortment of types of brick. Some protein foods will have lots of one type of brick, and other kinds of protein foods will have fewer of these and more of other types. The best and easiest way to ensure that you get a large range of bricks and enough of each kind of brick that you need to build and repair your body cells, is to mix the protein foods you take in at each meal.

Examples of plant sources of protein are bread, rice, spaghetti, and breakfast foods like porridge, Weetabix, and Shredded Wheat. These are all cereal products. Other plant sources are nuts, seeds, and pulses (peas and beans). If you consume a mixture of plant sources of protein (such as a cereal product with nuts, seeds, or pulses) then you will have a good mix of the kinds of building bricks (amino acids) that the body requires. This is just as beneficial as having animal protein. Plant proteins also have the advantage of being low in fat and high in fibre. What is more, protein from plants can be cheap and need not involve you in too much radical diet change. You just need to increase the frequency with which you eat protein from plant sources (and slightly decrease the amount of fatty animal proteins that you eat). Examples of good plant protein mixes are baked beans on toast; muesli (a mix which includes flakes of cereal and nuts); lentil or pea soup with bread rolls; vegetable curry (including lentils or peas) with rice.

If you usually think of products like bread or beans as sources of carbohydrate rather than protein, it is because much of the diet literature has emphasized this aspect of these foods. You are right in thinking that such products are carbohydrate sources too. However, this does not mean that the kinds of plant foods we have mentioned are bad or are to be avoided. They are so useful as low-fat sources of protein (and other nutrients too) that they are an important part of any food regime, including diets to reduce weight.

We have been generally talking about mixing different plant proteins but, of course, people generally mix plant with animal proteins in meals as part of a traditional way of eating. Examples are an animal protein (such as meat, fish, cheese, or egg) contained within a cereal product, bread, as a sandwich; breakfast cereal and milk; pizza (a flour base, the plant source of protein) with meat or fish and cheese topping; rice pudding; cheese on toast. There is absolutely no need, on any diet, to stop mixing protein sources in this way. It is a thoroughly good idea in order to obtain a wide range of nutrients. Difficulties only arise when dieters get it into their heads that only a certain source of protein is acceptable and therefore restrict the overall range. The tendency in the past has been to restrict or cut down on plant proteins and increase animal protein in the diet. Do not do this. If anything, increase plant protein and cut back on animal sources of protein, which are high in saturated fat. For example, if you feel like cheese on toast for lunch, rather than having a couple of slices of toast piled with cheese, have two slices of toast, one with just a moderate layer of cheese on top, and one with baked beans. If you have a glass of skimmed milk and a piece of fruit with this meal it will be even better. A good diet is a varied, mixed diet.

Carbohydrate and fibre

There are many different kinds of carbohydrate. Complex carbohydrate, or starch as many people term it, occurs in plant products such as bread, rice, spaghetti, flour, breakfast cereals (and cereals generally), potatoes, and in many vegetables. As well as starch, carbohydrate can occur naturally as simple sugars. For example, there is a sugar called lactose that is naturally present in milk; fruit sugar (fructose) and glucose occur together in many fruits. Generally speaking, where carbohydrate is taken in any of these forms, it is useful and is also accompanied by other nutrients. Meals for everybody, including slimmers, should contain such foods. Not only are such foods very nutritious, they also contain fibre. Generally it is recommended that there is more fibre in the diet to keep the gut working smoothly and efficiently. Fibre is the unabsorbed part of the food, a type of complex carbohydrate found in plant cell walls. To maintain fibre intake at an adequate level, it is best to have carbohydrate foods in 'whole' form. For example, eat the skins on jacket potatoes; use wholemeal flour in cooking; buy brown, wholemeal bread; use brown rice and brown spaghetti; take breakfast cereals that are not over-processed, such as Weetabix, Shredded Wheat, porridge oats, and sugar-free muesli. Plenty of fresh fruits and vegetables are also important. Dried fruits are especially high in fibre, as are pulses.

It is necessary, even if you are trying to lose weight, to maintain adequate carbohydrate and fibre levels. At each meal try to have at least one form of good carbohydrate such as we have mentioned above. Better still, have one form of complex carbohydrate (something starchy like rice or bread or pasta) plus a piece of fresh fruit. Be careful not to accompany your chosen carbohydrate with large quantities of fat. If you are eating carrots and potatoes with your meal, do not add a knob of butter or margarine. If you have chosen bread to make up sandwiches, use only the thinnest scrape of fat (preferably a polyunsaturated margarine or nothing at all). If you want potatoes with your meal, cook them more often as boiled or jacket potatoes rather than as chips. If you must have chips do them thick cut, as they absorb less fat that way. As you can see, the main mistake people make with carbohydrate is to use too much fat with it.

Another difficulty with carbohydrate food is that it is often over-refined. Sugar, the kind you buy in bags, is a highly refined form of sweetness, totally lacking in protein, minerals, vitamins, and fibre. Everyone, whether on a slimming diet or not, should reduce this kind of sugar to an absolute minimum. It can be surprisingly difficult to avoid, too, because it is added to so many foods and drinks. Biscuits, cakes, most fizzy drinks, squashes and fruit juices, sweets, chocolates, ice-cream, and jam all contain vast quantities of sugar. Savoury foods such as pickles, sauces, tinned vegetables, gravies, soups, and ready-made frozen meals often have sugar added. Read the labels on the foods you buy and you will be surprised at the number of hidden sources of refined sugar.

You can see why it is easy to be muddled about carbohydrate. Some diets have put all carbohydrate in the 'bad' category. This is a great pity. The thing to avoid or at least cut down on is refined sugar and the products that contain it. You will be more successful in this endeavour if you make sure you are not excessively hungry because of an over-restrictive diet. If your standard way of eating (or your slimming diet) includes a mix of proteins, complex carbohydrate, and fresh fruits at each meal, you are much less likely to eat large amounts of refined sugar or the products that contain it.

Fats

Some fat in the diet is essential to good health. However, not all fats are equally as good. The kind to use for preference is any variety which is labelled as polyunsaturated or as high in polyunsaturates. Where cooking fat is concerned, choose sunflower oil or safflower oil rather than blended vegetable oils or hard fats such as lard. This does not mean that you should fry everything in these 'good' oils and spread polyunsaturated margarine thickly on bread. Most people eat too much fat. It is actually not necessary to add fat to bread or vegetables or to cook with fat in order to obtain enough for good health. Many foods naturally contain sufficient of the kinds of fat needed for good health; you do not actually need to add extra. For example, the redder fishes like salmon, tuna, sardines, and kippers are good sources of polyunsaturated fat. Such essential fats are also found in some of the plant sources of carbohydrate we listed earlier (notably in nuts and seeds).

Despite the fact that they might not need it, most people like a little fat spread on bread or choose to have fried food occasionally. Do not have too much too often. Occasionally you might like to indulge yourself in a little olive oil (for example on salads) and this is fine as an occasional treat. This kind of fat is not a type high in polyunsaturates but, on the other hand, is not a hard saturated fat like lard or butter. Generally, if you are overweight, one of the easiest ways to get down to your ideal size is to cut fat intake right down. If you are the right weight already you could very probably still be healthier if you reduced your intake of saturated fats.

As well as obvious fat like butter, margarine, and oils there is much 'hidden' fat in many of the foods high in refined sugar, like biscuits, chocolate, and cake. So there is a doubly good reason for cutting down on these foods. Here are some other tips for reducing fat intake:

- Use skimmed or semi-skimmed milk rather than full-fat milk;
- Use cream less often on desserts and not at all in cooking;
- Have only three or four eggs a week;
- Buy more yogurt and less hard cheese;
- Eat less red meat and trim off the visible fat;
- Eat fewer fatty meat products such as sausages, meat pies, and burgers;
- Cut down on fatty snacks such as crisps;
- Use less pastry in cooking and buy fewer foods that incorporate pastry;
- Use less fat in cooking;
- If you are having a take-away meal such as fish and chips, leave some of the smaller, fattier chips usually found at the bottom of the bag. Leave some of the batter off the fish as well;
- If you are eating a pizza or pie do not feel duty-bound to finish off the whole thing. Leave a bit of the crust or the edge of the pizza base.

Remember that these are all *suggestions*, not commandments written in stone. You probably will not be able to cope with all of them without feeling deprived. The idea is gradually to introduce one or two of these ideas and see how you get on. If you absolutely love butter and hate polyunsaturated margarine, you would be foolish to make a rule to eat only margarine in future. Try some of the other suggestions instead or just try using slightly less butter than usual. Focus only on those things you fancy trying, at least at first. We show you how to set suitable goals in Chapter 8.

Vitamins and minerals: do you need more?

Severe shortage of vitamins and minerals is rare. However, any diet high in foods that contain few vitamins and minerals is likely to lead to some degree of illness. The average person, irrespective of weight, has too much refined sugar in their food. As sugar contains no vitamins and minerals, the calories supplied by food are 'empty', devoid of nutrients. If the person makes up for the deficit by eating extra nutritious food, then he or she might have an adequate amount of nutrients, but the high overall food and calorie intake will lead to obesity. Excess sugar really does cause many problems for lots of people.

Basically, if you follow the suggestions we have made earlier, you will obtain adequate supplies of vitamins and minerals. To summarize our suggestions for good nutrition:

- At each meal choose a mix of proteins from animal and plant sources; have low-fat protein sources more frequently;
- Carbohydrates should be in a 'natural', relatively unprocessed form, such as wholemeal bread, brown pasta and brown rice, or potatoes. Avoid refined sugar, whether white or brown;
- Have a piece of fruit with the meal;
- Keep fat to a minimum; choose polyunsaturated rather than saturated fat.

If you are eating enough of these kinds of food to maintain appropriate weight (or, if you are overweight, to lose weight slowly) then you should automatically be getting enough vitamins and minerals. There is no need to take supplements. Just to reassure you that a sensible eating plan will ensure that adequate nutrients are derived from the food, here is a brief outline of the topic.

Vitamins

Vitamins are present in the animal and plant sources of protein we outlined earlier, in fruits, in vegetables, and in some fats. Just a tiny quantity of each vitamin is necessary for the health and growth of body cells. Too much of some vitamins (notably A and D) can prove toxic: excess vitamin A or D can be difficult for the body to eliminate and therefore can act as a poison. It is not likely, however, that you will obtain too many vitamins from food and that this will prove problematic; the danger nearly always arises when a person takes too many vitamin tablets.

Vitamin A This is obtained from yellow or orange-coloured fruits and vegetables (such as apricots, melons, peaches, and carrots) and also from tomatoes, spinach, and peas. Good animal sources are the redder fish such as herring and sardines. It is also obtained in liver, kidney, dairy produce, and eggs. Margarine has vitamin A added, but this fat will not supply the protein available in the animal sources of vitamin A, or the vitamin C and fibre found in the fruit and vegetable sources of vitamin A.

Vitamin B There are a number of B vitamins. The main ones, B1, B2, and niacin, can be obtained from animal sources such as pork, liver, bacon, and plant sources like wholegrain cereals, wheatgerm, soya beans, and peanuts. As pork and bacon are both high in saturated fat, it is better to obtain B vitamins in the diet from other sources. Vitamin B6 is generally found in cereals, eggs, meat (liver is an especially rich source), and fish. Vitamin B12 is rather an odd vitamin as it is only obtained from animal sources (such as meat, milk, and eggs) and not at all from plant foods. It is absolutely essential, therefore, that vegans take vitamin B12 supplements. A deficiency in vitamin B12 may take many years to show, but it can prove fatal. However, this will only be a problem for those rare people who consume no animal products whatsoever. Vegetarians who consume eggs and milk should have no problem with obtaining enough vitamin B12.

Vitamin C Fresh fruit and vegetables, as most people know, are good sources of this vitamin. Frozen vegetables (such as peas and beans) generally retain their vitamin content well. They also have the advantage over most tinned varieties that they do not have salt or sugar added.

Vitamin D The body can manufacture its own vitamin D if exposed to sunlight. However, most people do not have the opportunity to obtain adequate vitamin D from this source. It is important to obtain enough of this nutrient because it is needed to facilitate the absorption of calcium in the diet. Certain susceptible groups such as pregnant women and children, who have a high calcium requirement, should do their utmost to ensure sufficient vitamin D is present in the diet. Red fish (such as herring, sardines, kippers, and salmon) are a reasonable, naturally occurring source of vitamin D. Eggs supply some of this nutrient, but not as much as red fish; because eggs are relatively high in saturated fat they should not be the main source of vitamin D. Margarine has this vitamin added, but again is not the preferred source because a good eating regime should not be too high in fat. Therefore red fish would seem to be the best major source of vitamin D, although vegetarians who do not eat fish need to rely on the other sources mentioned. Some varieties of skimmed milk have vitamins A and D added (read the labels) and can be a useful part of the diet.

These, then, are the major vitamins. There are others, but the above list represents the ones you need to be most concerned with. If your diet is good enough to supply enough vitamins A, B, C, and D from food and drink, other vitamin requirements will also be met automatically.

Minerals

There are many minerals needed by the body. Examples are iron, calcium, sodium, potassium, phosphorus, and magnesium. These are the inorganic elements in the diet, and although they are only needed in tiny amounts, they have very important functions. However, as with the vitamins, you will find that a sound diet with plenty of protein from various sources, good food derived from cereals, fruits and vegetables, should supply adequate minerals, with no need to take supplements.

The major minerals that most people are concerned with are iron and calcium. It is just possible that a diet too low in certain foods will produce iron and calcium deficiency. This is especially so for vulnerable groups (such as pregnant or lactating women, and children). A diet too high in refined sugar and fat will predispose to either obesity or shortage of nutrients, including minerals. It is extremely important, therefore, to follow the general principles on meal planning that we described earlier in the chapter. Here is some extra information that might help you plan a balanced eating regime.

Iron Many animal sources of protein are also good sources of iron. Particularly useful are liver, kidney, heart, beef, sardines, pilchards (red fish generally), and shellfish, including mussels and cockles. Iron from these sources is relatively well absorbed.

Iron is also present in plant sources of protein, such as peas, beans (including baked beans), lentils, spinach, porridge oats, wholemeal flour and wholemeal bread, soya flour and soya products, dry figs, apricots, sultanas, almonds, and brazil nuts. However, iron is far less readily absorbed from these plant sources than from animal sources. You also need to eat quite large quantities of these plant sources of iron in order to obtain enough. A few apricots or a slice of bread will not by themselves supply that much iron. You need to eat a reasonable portion of at least one plant source of iron at each meal if you do not eat meat or red fish. You can help your body use the iron from plant foods by eating fresh fruit (or any food or drink rich in vitamin C) along with the iron-rich food. Vitamin C is a great aid to helping your body utilize the iron present in your diet.

It is a good idea to vary your sources of iron. Simply to obtain all your supply of this mineral from one or two foods (say, dry figs or peas) would necessitate you eating an awful lot of these foods. Generally, if you have at least two or three slices of good wholemeal bread each day, and some other wholegrain cereal product, this will form a good base around which to design your meals, and add other iron-rich foods. If you have liver or a generous portion of a soya product at least once a week this will help. Soya flour is a good iron source that can be added to many foods (sauces, curries, bolognese, meat dishes like stews or cottage pie, bread or home-made cake mix, porridge). In fact, if you love cake and sweet things but you are concerned about the nutritional status of your diet, it is a good idea to experiment with making your own iron-rich 'health' cake. Use wholemeal flour instead of white. Add a little soya flour. Substitute polyunsaturated fat for saturated fat (and use less of it too). Add dried fruits like sultanas, dried dates, figs, apricots, and also chopped nuts. Grated apple or mashed banana can also add natural sweetness. Use skimmed milk and an egg for making the mixture moist; add a little apple juice too if you like. Do not bother adding sugar. A piece of this cake, with a glass of skimmed milk and a piece of fruit makes an easy but extremely nutritious meal. It is possible to cater for a sweet tooth and still have a healthy diet.

Calcium If you are having a reasonable amount of dairy

produce you are not likely to be short of calcium. A pint, or one-and-a-half pints of milk (preferably skimmed or semi-skimmed) each day provides a firm foundation for adequate calcium intake. However, some groups may need even more. Pregnant or lactating women, and children, might wish to either include more milk, or, to add to the variety, use yogurt frequently in cooking, or have it as a dessert, or have some cheese occasionally as well as milk.

There is also calcium in fish, and useful amounts can be obtained if the soft bones in some varieties of fish (like sardines, pilchards and salmon) are eaten along with the flesh. If you do not like the texture of the bones, put the fish in a food mixer; you will not even know the bones have been left in.

Fruits and vegetables contain acids that aid the absorption of calcium. This is an extra reason to have a combination of foods at a meal. Calcium is, in fact, present in some of the plant foods that contain the acids that aid absorption of this mineral. For example, some calcium is present in oranges. It can also be found in plant sources such as soya, brocolli, baked beans, almonds, brazil nuts, dried figs, and dried apricots. However these products tend not to be as rich in calcium as dairy products and red fish. An additional problem with plant sources of calcium is that calcium is not well absorbed when it is present without a rich protein source. Once again you can appreciate how important it is to have a mixed and varied diet.

Sodium There are various kinds of salt needed by the body but perhaps one of the most typical is sodium chloride (table salt). Salt is needed to maintain a good water balance in the body, and also for activity of muscle and nerve tissues. Generally we all have too much salt in the diet and our bodies have to work hard to excrete the excess. Salt occurs naturally in many foods and is added to even quite basic foods such as bread, so there is no need to add extra salt in cooking, or to food at the table. However, acquiring a taste for less salt may take time in order to become used to a low-salt taste. Luckily there are low-sodium salts available in supermarkets and chemists to help you in your endeavour. Potassium salt is sometimes used as a substitute, or mixed with sodium salt. Both of these are good ways to adjust to a better salt balance.

The functions of food

The body requires food for a number of reasons, which scientific study has only relatively recently revealed. Present knowledge about nutrition is probably just a very basic analysis of an extremely complex process. However, here is a very brief summary outlining the functions of food.

Food for fuel

In the same way that cars need fuel to help them move, we all need fuel to keep our bodies going. The carbohydrates (starches and sugars) and fats both provide fuel. If food intake is low the body starts to use its own sources of fuel, including fat stores (particularly important for the slimmer!). In extreme conditions where very little carbohydrate or fat is eaten, any protein intake can also be used as fuel. The body may also use its own lean tissue (muscle) as fuel when food intake is very low (such as when a person is on a crash diet) or when no food is taken at all.

Generally, though, it is carbohydrate and fat that provide fuel. The B vitamins are needed to release the energy from the fuel. Problems occasionally arise when individuals consume a great deal of refined sugar, because this is fuel food that has no B vitamins at all. This is an additional reason to ensure that carbohydrate foods are eaten in their wholegrain form (where there is an adequate supply of B vitamins).

Food for vitality

You need adequate oxygen supplied to body tissues in order to feel properly energetic and have a zest for life. If there is a slight deficiency of iron in the diet this adversely affects the amount of oxygen available to body tissues; you feel sluggish and tired, and this is usually termed anaemia. To prevent this condition it is important to ensure the diet contains enough iron, and enough vitamin C to help the absorption of iron from food. There are other causes of anaemia (for example one type of anaemia is due to lack of vitamin B12), but they are very much rarer than iron deficiency anaemia. As well as aiding iron absorption, vitamin C is also essential for the formation of connective tissue between cells.

A severe deficiency of vitamin C results in many symptoms, including listlessness, soft gums (even teeth falling out), and skin problems (symptoms of a disease called scurvy).

Food for repair and construction of new cells

Proteins are important for repair and construction of body cells. However, a high-protein diet need not be expensive, as we showed earlier. Calcium is also necessary for repair and construction of cells. Teeth and bones are largely composed of calcium and it is essential that enough of this mineral is present in the diet for them to remain strong. Vitamin D is necessary to aid the absorption of calcium from food. Vitamin A is also necessary for healthy growth of cells. It is required too for good eye function; difficulty in seeing in dim light may be a sign of vitamin A deficiency.

How about calories?

We have managed to get a fair way into this chapter on food and diet before mentioning that subject dear to a slimmer's heart, the calorific value of food. So, what is a calorie? It is not a vitamin, or a mineral, or a kind of sugar or fat. It is simply a measure of the energy supplied by *any* food or drink. This might be protein, fat, carbohydrate, or any combination of these three. They all can provide fuel in the diet and are therefore sources of energy. The same way we can measure length in feet and inches (or in metres), so we can measure the energy that food provides in calories. If your food and drink supplies you with exactly enough fuel to maintain your body's activities (the energy required to keep the vital functions going, and also for muscular work) then you will stay at a constant weight. If, on the other hand, you take in too few calories (that is, your diet supplies you with insufficient fuel to meet your energy requirements) you will draw on stored fuel. You will lose fat. Ideally, if you are overweight you will eat slightly less than is necessary to maintain a constant body weight. This need not mean drastically reducing food intake. Even a slight decrease, a sensible diet, will get you the results you want. Doing exercise, which requires extra fuel, will help burn off the body fat even quicker.

There are plenty of good, comprehensive calorie booklets on the market. If you feel like it, buy one and have a browse. It can be a real eye-opener to find how many calories there are in the foods you normally eat. The highest-calorie foods (in terms of number of calories per unit weight measurement) are all the fats. Concentrating on fat reduction in food is one of the best ways of ensuring a good weight loss. Foods like potatoes, rice, bread, pasta, vegetables, and fruit are all far lower in calories than fats (ounce for ounce). You need not be constantly totting up calories for everything that you eat (unless you want to of course), but do bear in mind the high calorie value of fat and keep it to a minimum.

Some ideas for meals

There are no hard and fast rules for planning healthy meals. There is not even an optimum number of meals or snacks that should be eaten each day. If you follow the recommendations we have made you can adapt your usual eating regime to make it more nutritious. You might also like to browse in the cookery section of your local library or bookshop. There are some excellent new books that focus on low-fat, low-sugar, low-salt, high-fibre recipes. However, what you primarily need are some very simple guidelines and ideas for meals. We finish this chapter by giving you examples of nutritious, well-balanced, easy meals. These are not at all original or exotic but are based on the ordinary things that most people tend to eat.

Breakfasts

Basically it is a good foundation to the day to include a glass of skimmed or semi-skimmed milk and a piece of fruit (or fresh fruit juice) with this meal. If you choose a cereal, use the milk on this; if you prefer something different, use the milk as a drink. Other good breakfast foods are:

- a wholegrain cereal such as Shredded Wheat, Weetabix, or porridge or sugar-free muesli;
- a bran cereal such as All-Bran or Bran Flakes;
- a slice of wholemeal toast with a *little* polyunsaturated margarine and one teaspoon of jam or marmalade;
- pre-soaked dried fruit such as apricots, prunes, or pears;
- a kipper and wholemeal bread;
- a slice of wholemeal toast topped with baked beans or an egg or a little cheese or sardines or pilchards;
- two well-grilled rashers of bacon with a tomato and a slice of wholemeal bread.

We have not always specified exact quantities of food. Eat according to appetite. If you are trying to lose weight limit yourself to the amounts necessary to attain your goal weight for the week (we explain this in detail in Part Two). Generally, though, all these breakfasts are likely to be low in calories. None of them come anywhere near the high calorific value of a big fried breakfast or even two or three slices of thickly buttered toast. Do not add fat to any of the food (except where we have specified it), and preferably omit salt too. If you absolutely must have sugar on cereal try to limit yourself to about one teaspoonful. Some of the things we have listed (such as Weetabix or baked beans) have sugar in them anyway so ideally you do not want to be adding even more sugar to breakfast meals. Try not to skip breakfast completely. Even if you are in a rush there should still be time for a glass of skimmed milk and a piece of fruit or fruit juice.

Main meals

Most people have two other meals besides breakfast. These might be of equal size or one small one and one larger one. Either way, the general guidelines for healthy eating stay the same, it is just the quantities of food that may be different. Here are some examples of simple yet highly nutritious meals.

Fish meals

- Prawn or salmon or tuna sandwich, fresh fruit, yogurt or skimmed milk;
- sardines or pilchards on toast with tomatoes, skimmed milk;
- kippers or mackerel, bread, yogurt, fruit;
- haddock, peas, potatoes, skimmed milk;
- cod, broccoli, grated cheese, tomatoes;
- prawn curry with peas and rice, skimmed milk;
- fish fingers, baked beans or peas, potatoes, grated cheese.

Meat meals

- Chilli con carne and rice (do not use much meat and use extra red beans), skimmed milk, fruit;
- spaghetti bolognese (again, use less meat and supplement with extra peas or soya or lentils)—sprinkle the meal with cheese and follow it with fruit;
- lean meat, jacket or boiled potatoes, any vegetables of choice, skimmed milk;

- corned beef and tomato sandwiches, yogurt;
- liver and onions, peas, carrots, potatoes, skimmed milk;
- meat and vegetable casserole or stew, skimmed milk;
- cottage pie with a thick potato topping, carrots, yogurt and fruit.

Cheese/egg meals
- Egg or cheese and tomato sandwiches, yogurt;
- egg or cheese on toast, fruit;
- jacket potato, grated cheese, sweetcorn;
- lentil or pea soup topped with grated cheese, bread, fruit;
- a two-egg omelette with baked beans or peas, bread, yogurt, fruit;
- cauliflower cheese, peas, bread;
- a liquid meal: a banana, skimmed milk, an egg and a little wheatgerm all whisked together into a milk-shake.

Vegan (strict vegetarian) meals
- Use soya meat or soya beans to make any of the meals listed under 'meat meals' that call for mince (for example a soya cottage pie or soya spaghetti bolognese);
- jacket potato or bread, salad (include peas or beans or sweetcorn), nuts, fruit;
- vegetable curry and rice, soya milk drink, fruit;
- sliced banana on toast sprinkled with chopped nuts and sultanas;
- baked beans on toast, fruit;
- nut spread and salad sandwiches, fruit;
- lentil or pea soup, bread, fruit.

With all the main meals listed, limit yourself to a very tiny amount of polyunsaturated fat for any cooking or spreading on bread. Add little or no salt or sugar to food. Always use brown (wholegrain) products rather than their refined, white counterparts.

You should choose a variety of foods and ring the changes with meals. Try to eat two or three meals a day. You can keep portions small enough to keep to your target weight. If you snack between meals (and most people do!) try to limit this to one or two snacks a day if you are trying to lose weight. Plan out something to eat during your vulnerable moments. Snacks can follow the same principle of low-fat, low-sugar eating as the main meals. Avoid becoming ravenously hungry. Food is there to keep you healthy and to enhance your enjoyment of life.

5

Your aim for exercise

It is impossible to avoid exercise. All human beings exercise every day of their lives. Getting dressed in the morning is exercise. Walking to the bathroom is exercise. Even lying in bed reading a newspaper, occasionally lifting your cup of tea to your lips, is exercise. You can consider exercise to be any movement you make.

If you are out of condition then exercise, or the movements you make, will cause you some degree of physical and possibly psychological distress. Is it difficult for you to lever yourself out of your chair? If the door bell goes, do you shuffle heavily along to answer it? Does climbing stairs leave you panting? Do daily chores tire you? Can you easily bend down to get your shoes on? Can you reach to wash your back in the bath? Is it difficult for you to carry two or three shopping bags? If you have any of these problems, you seriously need to consider extending your exercise capability by quite an amount. Even if you do not feel you have any of these kinds of difficulties, just how fit are you? Can you climb two or three flights of stairs, reasonably fast and taking the steps two at a time, and not end up breathless? Could you walk two miles in thirty minutes or run a mile in ten or twelve minutes? Are you reasonably supple? Do your shoulders creak if you swing your arms round in circles? Can you touch your toes while keeping your legs straight? How strong are you? Can you do five full press-ups from the floor (keeping your body and legs straight and supporting your weight on your toes and hands)?

Many individuals, once they leave school, do too little exercise to keep healthy and to maintain good weight control. Their exercise, in terms of the movements they make as part of everyday living, become increasingly difficult to perform. As running or walking any distance becomes uncomfortable, it is avoided more and more. A vicious circle therefore develops of doing less and less exercise. The less exercise you do, the more unfit you will become, and the harder everyday tasks will seem.

In addition, the loss of muscle tone will affect your looks. The unfit person will tend to be flabby and possibly fat. There will also be additional health problems associated with lack of exercise. If your leg muscles are inadequately used for walking or running you will be prone to develop varicose veins. You will be more likely to have high blood pressure and develop heart disease or have a stroke. Your muscles, joints, and bones will be weaker than they should be. Your face will be more likely to have a dull complexion, with podgy, sagging cheeks and double chin. Your metabolic rate will fall; eating just average amounts of food will tend to make you fat. You will probably be less able to cope with the pressures of life; the ability to cope and be relaxed does not come easily to a body that indulges in too little physical activity and is unhealthy. Too little exercise during the day and you will find it difficult to have a good night's sleep.

You can see that there are plenty of reasons to maintain a reasonable level of exercise. You next need to decide on the kinds of exercise you might choose to do.

Three different kinds of exercise: for stamina, for suppleness, and for strength

Stamina

Another equally good word for this is endurance exercise. Stamina or endurance refers to your capacity to keep up a certain level of sustained exercise. If you are low in stamina you will have lost your ability to get through the day without becoming over-tired. An ordinary shopping trip will leave you weary. You will not be able to play much with the children (or anyone else for that matter!) without becoming weary. You will get breathless easily.

If you want to get the most out of life you need to maintain a certain level of muscular stamina. Exercises that increase stamina are those that require you to breath slightly more heavily than usual for a prolonged period of time (say, an exercise session of thirty minutes or so). Here are some good exercises to increase stamina:

- brisk walking;
- jogging;
- swimming;
- cycling;
- any sport with sustained activity which increases pulse rate for prolonged periods.

It is important that you do your chosen exercise at a pace that makes you slightly breathless and increases your heart rate, but not so much that you cannot maintain the exercise for at least twenty or thirty minutes. A brisk walk or jog for half-an-hour will do much more to build stamina than a twelve-second sprint.

Obviously there are many sports that involve moving around faster than normal. To be able to play most competitive games well you need stamina; indulging in sport on a regular basis builds stamina. A good game of tennis, badminton, hockey, netball, or football, for instance, all involve a great deal of running over a prolonged period of time. Do be careful if you are unused to sport. Do not try too hard too soon. This is especially true if you are playing a sport such as squash, where an extremely high level of stamina is needed right from the very beginning. It can be dangerous to over-exert yourself greatly at the beginning of your fitness programme. It is much better to build up endurance levels gradually and gently over a period of weeks and months. That way you will increase stamina and also build a better cardiovascular system. Your heart will be healthier and you will be far less likely to have a heart attack or stroke when you get older than someone who has exercised very little during their life. Finally, it is worth remembering that exercise to increase stamina will boost metabolic rate. If you have excess fat you will burn it off quicker. If you are not too fat you will be able to eat more and not put on weight.

Suppleness

This kind of exercise, as the name implies, involves stretching, bending and twisting kinds of movement. Most standard kinds of exercise routines and work-outs contain many suppleness exercises. Examples are circling your arms around from your shoulders; toe-touching; standing upright then bending your body sideways to the left then right; lying on the floor then raising each leg as high in the air as possible (keeping the leg straight). If you do such exercises fast and you repeat them, and manage to become breathless in the process for a twenty to thirty-minute period, you have combined your suppleness exercise with stamina exercise. Aerobics classes (or 'pop-mobility') or exercise tapes for home use, can be a splendid way to build endurance and suppleness when done on a regular basis. However, do remember that if suppleness exercise is done without it inducing heavier breathing and an increased heart-rate (for example, yoga) this will do very little for increasing your stamina.

Many of the sports we mentioned as being good for stamina also require you to stretch and swing and twist your limbs and torso and are therefore good for suppleness also. Most racket games are good examples, as are some ball games such as football. Swimming is an excellent all-round sport. Exercise that requires a limited sort of movement, such as walking or jogging, may be excellent for stamina but is not useful for suppleness.

Strength

Strong muscles are not necessarily big and bulky muscles. It is necessary for everyone, male or female, to maintain adequate muscle strength. Weak muscles will give you a flabby shape and bad posture. Strengthening your muscles need not make them bigger, but firm and taut. You will have a better body shape. You will be able to do general chores easier. If you have babies or young children you will be able to lift them with little effort. If you strengthen the muscles in your back you will be far less likely to damage your back or suffer from chronic back pain. Strong abdominal muscles will prevent you from having a 'pot belly'.

Perhaps the most obvious way to build strength is by training with weights. Expert advice from a local gym or sports centre can be very helpful when you are starting with weights. If you lift heavy weights and you lift in the wrong way, you can obviously do yourself damage. Lifting very heavy weights can also raise your blood pressure considerably for a short time. The best way to train with weights, for the average person, is to do repetitions of movements using relatively light weights. This builds stamina as well as strength. Once you have obtained some professional advice on weight training you can obtain small weights (such as hand weights) quite cheaply for use at home (if you do not have the time or inclination to travel to a gym to exercise).

There are other ways of building strength besides lifting weights. Some sports magazines and shops sell weighted strips of material that you can wear around your wrists or ankles whilst doing other exercise (such as suppleness exercises or when running). This will help increase muscle strength.

There are relatively simple exercises to build strength. Examples of which most people have heard are press-ups, stomach curls, and leg lifts. With press-ups you lie on your stomach on the floor and, keeping your back straight, you push your body upwards so that your arms are straight and your body is supported on your toes and hands. For stomach curls you lie on your back on the floor, bend your knees upwards slightly (while keeping your feet on the floor), then lift your head and shoulders a few inches off the floor (do not use your hands or arms to support your weight). Hold this position for a few seconds then let your shoulders and head go back slowly to the floor. The third exercise, leg lifts, is to help strengthen your back. You start by lying on your stomach with your legs out straight behind you and your arms straight at your sides. Your hands should be under your thighs. You lift your head and arch your back and, at the same time, you lift your right foot as far off the ground as you can (while keeping your leg straight). You then return to the lying flat starting position, and then go on to repeat the exercise using the other leg.

These exercises can easily be incorporated into an exercise routine, with each exercise repeated a number of times. Indeed, many exercise tapes or aerobics sessions contain muscle-strengthening exercises of the sort we have just described. If such exercises are repeated quickly enough to cause you to become breathless for a prolonged period, you will be building stamina too.

Some sports also build strength. It should come as no surprise that cycling builds leg strength. You can feel the leg muscles really hardening as you pedal hard up a hill. Swimming builds strength, stamina, and suppleness. Yoga may not do much for stamina, but it can be excellent for suppleness and also relatively good for strength.

Which exercise should you choose?

Before the days of household appliances like washing machines and vacuum cleaners, and before motorized transport, people were more likely to obtain plenty of exercise in normal day-to-day activity. They did not need special fitness regimes. More people had physically active jobs. Looking after a household involved strenuous activity. Modern houses have so many labour-saving devices that it is difficult for the person at home to have adequate exercise by doing chores, cooking, and looking after a family. Jobs outside the home tend to be more sedentary. Travel is often by car, bus, or train. Even within the work environment you can often take a lift rather than use stairs.

You could probably become far more healthy by the simple expedient of 'going back in time' in terms of some of your daily activity. You could use a bike, walk, or run rather than use a car, bus, or train. You could do more domestic tasks by hand rather than using electrically operated gadgets. However, this approach has too many problems to be appealing. After the luxury of labour-saving devices it is just too tedious to go back to the old ways. Also, this is not the most efficient way to build up and maintain a reasonable level of physical fitness. You actually only need to plan three or four exercise sessions a week in order to become fit. Each session should ideally be about thirty minutes long. Of course, you can always do more but it is encouraging to know that you can reap the benefits of exercise in just ninety minutes a week.

As with healthy diet, healthy exercise requires an appropriate balance of different components. You need adequate and appropriate exercise to build strength, suppleness, and stamina. You can pick from the examples we have described. However, this does not necessarily mean that you need to do lots of different kinds of exercise. Find the right exercise menu to suit your personality and life-style. For example, if you like swimming, this exercise is good for strength, stamina, and suppleness; three swimming sessions a week will make you considerably fitter.

If you are the stay-at-home type you might like to choose an exercise book or tape that covers strength and suppleness exercises of the kind we have described. Videos are often available of exercise routines so you can see exactly what you should be doing. If your exercise session is fairly strenuous and makes you pant a bit (and takes at least twenty minutes) your stamina will also increase. If you think you will get bored with the same kind of exercise, experiment with different types. For example, you could jog or walk briskly for a mile or two for one exercise session; use an exercise tape for another session; and participate in something different like weight-training, or cycling, or a ball or racket game, for a third session in the week. A basic principle is to try out the things you think you are most likely to enjoy and to incorporate them into your routine on a long-term basis. There are gadgets available to make exercise more fun. You can buy weights to use at home. Exercise bikes and rowing machines are becoming more popular. Even a very basic thing like a skipping rope is a cheap but good aid to exercise (building stamina especially). There are all sorts of fashionable exercise outfits to wear while doing your chosen exercise. Go to some trouble to make a proper start to your programme. If you invest a little money and buy, for example, an exercise tape or jogging shoes or a leotard or a piece of exercise equipment, you will have added incentive for the start of your fitness schedule.

It could be that you are a very sociable, competitive sort. Obviously you might be better joining a club to participate in sport. You can also combine or alternate these outings with at-home exercise sessions if you wish. No matter what your chosen activity (dance, aerobics, yoga, weight-lifting, tennis and so on) there is a good chance that some class or club will be available near you and that you can join. If not, you can always start your own small group with one or two friends.

Finding the time to exercise

It is possible that you might find it difficult at first to make time for exercise. You should remember that adequate physical exercise is essential to good health. It affects the quality of your everyday existence. It will help you lead a long and productive life. Exercise is just as important as other little extras you fit into your routine. You would not dream of not bathing, washing your face, or washing your hair. If you can find time for basic personal hygiene you can find time for exercise. However, it may take a little planning at first. You need to consider your present life-style. If you are busy at home or out at work (and perhaps you have others to look after as well) it can be hard to envisage any free time. But families can join in with exercise too. For example, children love to join in with what they see as adult pastimes. If you change into a leotard and exercise, young children will want to copy you and participate. It will become a game for them. Family walks can be fun; taking a good walk to the shops can be fitted into most routines. The occasional trip to a swimming pool is a real treat for most families. If you are out at work, a brisk walk at lunch-time might be possible. Plan out some ordinary ways to increase exercise as part of your usual routine. Take stairs rather than lifts or escalators; do not trudge up them as if you were mounting Everest but go as briskly as you can. If you are walking anywhere, even around the house, walk more quickly. Make a conscious effort to speed up activity in this way.

You need to consider your exercise programme in the context of other things going on in your life. Many good exercise programmes stop when life and the usual routine starts to get chaotic or change for some reason. For example, what happens when you go on holiday for a few weeks, or you are bedridden with influenza, or you change job or move house? Ideally, provided you are not ill, you can continue with some exercise, even if it is less than you are used to. If you cannot manage anything, you can always just enjoy a short break and plan a date and a strategy for the return to your exercise routine. Never think that you have blown your exercise schedule so you may as well not bother going back to it. You might occasionally need to change your exercise programme to fit in with different needs or different time constraints but it is essential that you maintain an adequate level of physical fitness. You will be better able to cope with the stresses and strains of life; your self-esteem, your psychological and physical competence, should benefit.

Part II

How to achieve easy, effective weight control

5

Willpower explained

Many people think of [illegible] [illegible] [illegible]. You [illegible] [illegible] [illegible] [illegible] [illegible] or [illegible] [illegible] [illegible] [illegible] what you [illegible] [illegible] [illegible] [illegible] [illegible] [illegible] [illegible] of [illegible] [illegible] [illegible] [illegible] [illegible] personality and behaviour is not [illegible] [illegible] people are amazingly adap[illegible] [illegible] [illegible] characteristics that [illegible] [illegible] [illegible] [illegible] [illegible] have [illegible] [illegible] [illegible] [illegible]

For example, [illegible] [illegible] [illegible] [illegible] [illegible] [illegible] [illegible] [illegible] with [illegible] [illegible] [illegible] to become [illegible]. Anxious [illegible] [illegible] [illegible] [illegible] [illegible]. And people [illegible] [illegible] their own intake [illegible] [illegible] appropriate [illegible] [illegible] [illegible] [illegible] shape.

[illegible] [illegible] [illegible] life's way you pick up little techniques. [illegible] your behaviour, get yourself [illegible] [illegible] [illegible] just so happens that some [illegible] techniques without too much [illegible] because of circumstances and the people they [illegible] [illegible] some individuals [illegible] [illegible] [illegible] [illegible] [illegible] [illegible] [illegible] [illegible] [illegible]

If you want to be strong-willed you have [illegible] [illegible] that people [illegible] [illegible] [illegible]

6

Will-power explained

Many people think of personality characteristics as virtually unchangeable. You are either strong-willed or you are not. You are an optimistic type, or you are not. You succeed in what you set out to do, or you are someone who most often fails or falls short of your target. Interestingly, this view of personality and behaviour is not strictly accurate. Human beings are amazingly adaptive. Many of the so-called personality characteristics that people manifest, and many of the habits they have acquired, are subject to modification. Psychology makes a great deal of this malleability of behaviour and has developed a technology designed to help people overcome behavioural difficulties and overcome habit problems. Hence, psychology in practice has many facets. For example, shy people can learn to become more socially skilled. Individuals with specific fears and phobias can learn to become unafraid. Anxious clients can be taught to cope with stress. And people with weight problems can learn to control their food intake and adjust their energy expenditure by appropriate exercise, in order to attain physical fitness and a slim shape.

You are not born with strong or weak will-power. Along life's way you pick up little techniques that help you control your behaviour, get your own way, become strong-willed. It just so happens that some people get taught or pick up techniques without too much problem (because of circumstances and the people they interact with and learn from) but some individuals simply do not get exposed to the right experiences to learn these things in quite the same way.

If you want to be strong-willed you have to learn a few basic things that people with good self-control and will-power have managed to pick up. You will be able to tackle and succeed in almost anything provided you set about the problem in the right way. It is not necessary to try to change your mental characteristics directly, to somehow think yourself better controlled. Concentrate instead on studying your own behaviour, your interactions with your environment; by working on external factors in this way you will be able to work out practical strategies to succeed, and strong will-power will appear to come about automatically without you having to work on it directly. Goals are much easier to attain if they are broken down into small steps. Reward yourself for success. You should look, too, at the circumstances in the past in which you have achieved some modicum of success, and analyse why this occurred. Think, too, about the circumstances under which you cannot keep to your resolves, and analyse exactly what it is that makes you behave the way you do.

Consider your past attempts at weight control. Did you use diet, exercise, or both? If you failed, what were the reasons that you failed? Do not look to internal, mental explanations. A weak will is not the answer. If you failed it must be because of complex interactions with your environment. Success was too difficult to attain for practical, identifiable reasons. In trying to pinpoint these reasons, it will help if you think of diet attempts in three distinct parts.

The first concerns antecedent events, that is, those things that happen and act as 'triggers' for specific behaviours. Some stimuli in the environment will help you diet, and some will have just the opposite effect. For example, imagine the situation where you have been on a strict, very low calorie diet for a month or so. You lost a fair amount of weight to begin with but in the last week you have only dropped 1 lb (0.4 kg) and you are disappointed with progress. You quarrelled with your spouse on the way out to the shops and you are feeling angry. You are also really hungry. You go into a café where the sight and smell of freshly baked Danish pastries hits you squarely in the face as you walk through the door. You may have only intended to have a small black coffee but given all the antecedent events (that is, the things we have described leading up to walking into the café), the probability is high that you will break the diet. A saint would break a diet under these circumstances. You need to consider those antecedent events that prompt you to break a diet, and then think about which of these things you can avoid or change in some way.

The second part of your review of previous diet attempts involves a close look at your weight control behaviour. What diets have you tried? Which did you succeed most with and which did you fail badly with? What food do you eat normally, and what do you eat when you diet? What do you like to eat?

The third area you should consider involves the consequences of your weight control behaviour. Do you actually lose weight when you try to diet? For how long does it stay off? Do you reward yourself in any way for your success? Do you punish yourself or feel guilty if you fail? When you stop a diet is it because you plan to, or do you go suddenly into a binge? If you do over-eat, how long does this last; an hour, a day, a week?

These three parts of your analysis—Antecedent events, Behaviour, and Consequences—can be termed the ABC, or basic units that you need to consider if you want to change your behaviour in the way you wish. To give you a better idea of how these three areas can contribute to self-control and ability to succeed with weight control, we will next look at each of them in some detail.

The 'A' of behaviour change: antecedent events

We have just given you an example of a typical dieter's antecedent events, leading to the breaking of the diet. We will take each of the main triggering events and look at them in more detail. By understanding this example you will be better able to set about understanding your own situation and the things that control your own dieting behaviour. The events that triggered our dieter into breaking the diet were:

1. A weight loss of only 1 lb (0.4 kg) in the previous week (less than expected for the effort put in). The feeling that goes with this is disappointment and frustration.
2. A quarrel with someone close. The feeling of anger and hurt now gets added to the disappointment and frustration.
3. A general state of hunger (following little or no breakfast allowed on the restrictive diet).
4. Going into a location (a café) associated with food and with pleasant, comforting eating experiences in the past.
5. Smelling and seeing Danish pastries, and seeing other customers in the café eating and apparently enjoying food.

There are ways of coping with all these five kinds of events. First, consider the situation where weight loss is not as good as expected. This must happen to most dieters at some time or another. The situation is difficult to cope with unless you rehearse in advance some useful strategies. You can try to rationalize your low weight loss. Why did it occur? Is it that you may actually have lost fat but the loss may not show much on the scales because you are retaining water. Did you have a salty meal and therefore drink more? Or (for a woman) is your period due and that is causing you to weigh more than usual? Perhaps you ate more than you realized the previous week? On the other hand you may be expecting too fast a weight loss. Weight is very quickly lost in the first week or so of most diets, but slows down somewhat after that. Perhaps your expectations are not realistic and you should be happier with a slower weight loss. It really does not matter if you do not lose weight every week. Try not to regain weight, and go for an overall loss by the end of each month. If you look closely at the situation and try to understand why it happened, you will be able to adopt an objective approach that stops you feeling anguish, prevents you from feeling a failure. This is very important because once you start to perceive yourself in negative terms you will probably start to act in a negative way, being quarrelsome and finally looking to food for comfort.

The second antecedent event, quarrelling with another person, often follows closely on a feeling of disappointment and personal failure. If you are feeling slightly down, the smallest things are likely to irritate you. Even if the quarrel is not started by you at all, you will be less able to cope and respond appropriately if you are already slightly under the weather. Try to keep your interactions with others as a separate issue from dieting problems. If you know you cannot deal with an upsetting confrontation, try to put it off for a short while until you feel calmer. Take your mind off negative things by dwelling on something positive and interesting that does not involve eating. Try relaxation, try yoga, try a long walk, try reading a magazine, having a bath—*anything* that you personally enjoy and that enhances your sense of well-being.

In our example, the dieter is in a fairly negative mental state and is also extremely hungry. If you fail to lose weight as you feel you should, it is temping to cut down on food even more to get better results. This rarely works. Severe hunger usually leads to extreme bingeing. If you are sincerely dieting in a way that has led you to lose weight in the past, just stick with the same regime for a further week or two. You should find the weight will drop quite acceptably. Any good weight loss regime should not lead to extreme hunger; it should be so easy that you can stick with the diet until all the weight is off.

The final events that lead our dieter to break the diet are quite concrete, namely, walking into a café, seeing and smelling the pastries, and seeing other people happily enjoying them. If you realize that you are especially susceptible at some particular time it is foolish to place yourself directly in temptation's way. If you think you could well get out of control you can avoid triggering stimuli as much as possible. Do not go into cafés, browse in cake shops, linger over the chocolate counter, or bake a batch of biscuits. You will succumb to temptation, and probably more than once. Dieters do not typically break their diet by having just one small biscuit, or one square of chocolate, or one tiny cake. They have the whole packet of biscuits, or three or four bars of chocolate, or, with our example in the café, a full fried breakfast followed by a Danish pastry. So, avoid those places or situations that are likely to make you want to over-eat. Strengthen your motivation to stay with your chosen weight control regime. Again, you must work out what suits you best. Good examples of activities to maintain motivation are collecting inspiring dieting case histories from slimming magazines; going out to buy a dress one size smaller than your present size; looking at charts and graphs that show good overall weight loss over a period of time. You might also allow yourself one small indulgence with food now and again. If you are totally fed up, *one* extra bar of chocolate or cake or any one single luxury item is not going to set you back to square one. Plan and control your chosen indulgence. Perhaps you might even feel like not dieting for one or two days. Decide on the time off the diet, plan proper balanced meals with the odd luxury for this period, and do not go wild and regain your lost weight. Just aim to stay where you are until the tough period is over and you can recommence your weight loss regime. Do not feel guilty about giving yourself a little time off occasionally like this. Continue to eat nutritious food and enjoy it.

Once you begin to understand some of the antecedent events that control your own eating behaviour you will be able to plan out a positive approach, by working out those antecedent events most likely to lead to success. Some common strategies likely to lead to success are listed below:

1. Restrict the locations in which you keep food (there is no need for food in bedrooms, food in your pockets, or in your handbag, for example).
2. Decide on set places or locations to eat (say, the dining

room table). This should prevent certain other locations, like the chair in front of the television, becoming a cue to start eating.

3. Keep a good stock of nutritious foods available: do not fill your cupboards with sweets, biscuits, chocolates, and other high-fat, high-sugar foods of this nature.
4. Plan to eat often enough that you do not get extremely hungry and lose control.
5. Try to eat slowly and really savour your food at meals so that you feel satisfied and therefore less likely to snack later on.

The 'B' of behaviour change: behaviour directly related to weight control

Consider how you normally eat. If you are not on a diet what is your pattern of eating behaviour? At what times do you eat? Do you have rigid meal times and snack in between; is eating planned or very haphazard? Do you eat when it is a certain time, or do you eat when you are hungry? How do you eat? Is eating a leisurely process? How long does it take you to consume a meal? How would you eat a bar of chocolate? This may seem like an odd question but there is quite some difference between eating styles, especially eating related to what is often viewed as 'naughty' food. For example, would you cut the chocolate into pieces and eat them slowly, perhaps accompanied by a drink? Or would you eat the chocolate very quickly without thinking or even looking much at it at all? Would you save some until later? Perhaps your first bar is simply a prelude to many more? What kinds of savoury food do you eat? Do you serve yourself large portions? Would you eat other people's left-overs? Would you normally eat a dessert after a large meal? Just think about the answers to such questions for now. Later we show you how to monitor your usual eating behaviour in order to obtain a 'baseline'. A baseline in this case is simply a complete record, a type of diary, of your usual eating behaviour. This forms a base against which to compare future progress.

As well as your normal eating think about your past attempts at weight control. List every kind of diet you remember trying. How long did each last? How much weight do you remember losing on each, and for how long did it stay off? Did you enjoy any of these diets, and if so, why? What kinds of food do you like to be allowed on a diet? If your weight has gone up and down over the last year (or ten years!) try to remember when and why it was up or down. What were the significant events happening in your life at the time? Are there any themes you can pick out? Look at your past history to learn lessons about your own behaviour. If you feel you are a mess do not worry. By setting realistic goals and tackling your weight control programme in easy steps you will learn to control your eating behaviour in a way that pleases and satisfies you.

The 'C' of behaviour change: consequences related to weight control attempts

The consequences of dieting generally fall into two distinct categories: those you dearly wish would happen, and those that actually do happen. What you want is to find yourself slim and attractive after a time on an easy, satisfying diet. You want the weight to stay off and you also want to be able to eat a reasonable amount of food after the diet without putting on weight. What actually does happen, in most cases, is that either you do not lose the weight in the first place, or, if you do, it is on a difficult diet and when it finishes you get fat once again.

It is possible to programme additional consequences into your weight control regime to strengthen your motivation and to increase the probability that what you want to happen actually does take place. The problem with weight loss is that it takes a long time to get what you want. It is necessary, therefore, to arrange additional, pleasing consequences along the way.

When people join a slimming club they are, in effect, giving themselves a boost, a social reward for slimming. Meeting others in the same position, having a chat with friends about dieting endeavours, these things help to maintain motivation. You need to consider what consequences, what additional motivating events or rewards you can use to keep you going. Get your partner, friends, and family to sponsor you if this is possible. If you cannot do this, you could put aside a certain amount of money as a reward for each time the scales register a drop in weight. Think about tangible gifts you might buy yourself.

Weight loss is itself a rewarding consequence, but because you need to lose a fair amount of weight before it is really noticeable in terms of body shape, you will probably require extra rewards to keep you going. If you mark your weight on a graph or chart this should provide a clear and rewarding sign of progress over a period of weeks and months.

Write out a list of rewards. Make sure they are practical and are within your budget (or your spouse's or friend's budget!). Make rewards contingent upon quite small amounts of progress. Rewards need to be fairly frequent. Obviously you have to work within certain financial constraints. If money is a problem rewards can be built around things you like doing. For example, if you enjoy a trip into town or to a cinema, museum or art gallery, save it up as a reward for good progress. Another possibility is to let yourself off doing jobs you do not like as a reward for making good progress. Preferably you can arrange for someone else to do these jobs for you. Be imaginative in making up your reward scheme. Make specific the goals you need to attain in order to earn each reward. Write it all down—this forms what is termed a 'contingency contract'. Looking through this contract at what goodies you can earn is in itself an act to strengthen motivation and keep you on track.

Notice that we have only mentioned reward, not punishment. Do not attempt to punish yourself for not making adequate progress. The fact that you have not made the progress you aimed for is punishing enough without adding more aversive consequences. If you fail to make a goal, analyse why. Consider what you can do to avoid this in the future. Treat this as a learning experience.

Finally, you can plan ahead and continue with some sort of contingency contract when you have attained your ideal weight. There is no reason why you should not have a weekly reward for remaining the same weight, at least for a few months after you have attained your ideal shape. For some people, staying the same weight is just as difficult as losing weight.

Exercise

We have talked about antecedent events, behaviour, and consequences as applied to eating behaviour and dieting. Exercise has not been included in this because too few people have a history of exercise attempts in the same way as they have diet attempts. For most slimmers, exercise is a non-issue. This is rather a pity, for the reasons we explained in Chapter 5. You must consider exercise as a top priority for the future. Include exercise as a part of your contingency contract. Programme rewards for doing certain exercises or sports each week. Think about the antecedent events most conducive to exercise, and the rewards most likely to maintain it.

Practical aids

To maintain motivation and strengthen will-power you can use simple, practical aids to monitor progress and highlight the changes that have happened while you have been losing weight.

Use a camera

We recommended that you have photographs taken when we gave you advice on assessing your shape in Chapter 3. If this idea appeals to you, you can go on to have your photograph taken every four to six weeks during your weight loss campaign. Always wear clothes to reveal your shape when having these taken, and adopt more or less the same poses. Keep an album especially for these pictures, and record the date and your weight under the photographs.

Weighing scales

Do you have scales with which to weigh yourself? What are they like? If they are years old and rusty they are probably not much good. You must know the kind of thing we mean. You get on them slowly and they register one weight; if you jump on them with gusto they register something quite different. In fact, you can just get on and off them a few times and they never seem to register the same thing twice! We would strongly recommend that if your scales are unreliable you should banish them to the bin and invest in some new ones. Digital scales are quite popular and have the benefit that you do not have to interpret just which tiny little weight line seems to be indicated as your weight.

Accurate weighing will be an essential part of your new campaign. You will not have to record every tiny thing you eat or work out calories but it is important that each day you weigh yourself if you possibly can. Weigh at the same time and under the same conditions each day. We recommend first thing in the morning, before breakfast, undressed, and having visited the lavatory! You will need to record your daily weight. If you do not have scales and cannot afford them, try to borrow some, or find your nearest public scales and visit them as often as you can.

You may be a little surprised to learn that we want you to weigh each day. Most experts recommend once a week because it takes this long for any real loss to show. While this is true, we want you to feel in control of your weight and to be able to interpret the minor fluctuations that occur from day to day. If you weigh slightly more one morning than the next, why should that be? Did you have a salty meal the day before that caused you to retain water, or was the last meal of the day unusually late? Are you constipated at all or (for women) is your period due?

A happy thought is that a gain of 2–3 lb (1 kg) in a day is extremely unlikely to be due to fat alone. To add 2 lb (just under 1 kg) of body fat in a day you need to eat about 7000 calories in addition to the normal amount you need to maintain body weight (about 2000 calories). You are extremely unlikely to eat this amount—some 9000 calories—in one day. Most bars of chocolate are about 300 calories per bar. So, if you ate, say, thirty Mars bars in a day you might just put on 2 lb (1 kg) of fat. Most cakes (including cream cakes) are about 300–500 calories each. So you would need to eat between eighteen and thirty cakes to add 2 lb (1 kg) of fat in a day. We put this to you as an answer to all slimmers who say they only need to look at a single cake or bar of chocolate to put on a substantial amount of fat. It is impossible. Even a normal 2000 calories-worth of meals in a day would need to be supplemented by fourteen cakes at 500 calories each, or around twenty bars of chocolate, to add 2 lb (1 kg) of fat in one day. It is most unlikely that you would do this!

However, you might quite easily eat *slightly* too much (an intake amounting to 500 calories) each day. Over 30 days this is 30 × 500 = 15 000 calories in excess. This would be 4 lb (just under 2 kg) of fat added to your body; you would be putting on around 1 lb. (0.4 kg) of fat a week. If you do not weigh yourself for a month, finding a 4 lb (about 2 kg) gain might be something of a surprise. If you do not weigh for a year and you eat just an extra 500 calories each day during that time, you will have put on a full 48 lb (21.8 kg); rather a nasty shock! Generally, therefore, we recommend that you weigh yourself each day. You will not see vast amounts of fat lost in a day, but you will come to understand how your behaviour relates to your body weight, and you will also avoid getting a horrendous shock when you step on the scales. You can write your weight in a diary or on a chart or graph and see progress develop in the right direction over time. You will be in control.

Charts, graphs, a diary

You will need to write down certain things like a list of goals for food change and exercise, interesting recipes, a list of rewards (perhaps as part of a contingency contract), and your daily weight. A basic diary will help to get you organized and you will be able to keep track of your aims on any particular week.

A graph or chart of weight can be useful. You need to interpret your list of daily weights in order to see if, over a month or so, it is going up, down or staying the same. One way of doing this is to count the number of days in any month where you were at or below a certain weight. For example, look at Table 2. You can see that in January this person weighed 9 st 8 lb (60.8 kg) for eight days, 9 st 7 lb (60.3 kg) for twelve days, 9 st 6 lb (59.9 kg) for five days, 9 st 5 lb (59.4 kg) for five days, and 9 st 4 lb (59.0 kg) just once.

In February our slimmer was never 9 st 8 lb (60.8 kg), was 9 st 7 lb (60.3 kg) for only six days, 9 st 6 lb (59.9 kg) for five days, 9 st 5 lb (59.4 kg) for six days, 9 st 4 lb (59.0 kg) for six days, 9 st 3 lb (58.5 kg) for five days and 9 st 2 lb (58.1 kg) just once (a weight not attained at all in January).

Things get even better in March. Our slimmer is never above 9 st 4 lb (59.0 kg), spends most days at 9 st 3 lb (58.5 kg), and goes as low as 9 st 0 lb (57.2 kg).

In April, our slimmer reaches 8 st 11 lb (55.8 kg), is often at 9 st 1 lb (57.6 kg), and never goes above 9 st 3 lb (58.5 kg).

Table 2 A daily weight record

	Weight			
Day	January st lb	February st lb	March st lb	April st lb
1	9 8	9 6	9 3	9 0
2	9 7	9 5	9 4	9 1
3	9 8	9 5	9 4	9 1
4	9 8	9 6	9 2	9 0
5	9 7	9 6	9 3	9 1
6	9 8	9 6	9 4	9 3
7	9 8	9 7	9 3	9 2
8	9 8	9 7	9 3	9 2
9	9 7	9 6	9 3	9 2
10	9 7	9 7	9 2	9 1
11	9 7	9 7	9 3	9 0
12	9 8	9 7	9 3	9 0
13	9 7	9 5	9 2	8 13
14	9 7	9 5	9 3	8 13
15	9 6	9 5	9 2	9 0
16	9 7	9 4	9 2	9 1
17	9 7	9 5	9 2	9 1
18	9 6	9 4	9 3	9 1
19	9 7	9 3	9 3	9 1
20	9 8	9 4	9 2	9 0
21	9 7	9 4	9 3	9 0
22	9 7	9 3	9 1	9 0
23	9 6	9 2	9 1	9 1
24	9 5	9 3	9 0	9 0
25	9 6	9 3	9 1	8 13
26	9 5	9 4	9 0	8 12
27	9 5	9 3	9 2	8 13
28	9 4	9 4	9 1	8 12
29	9 5		9 0	8 11
30	9 5		9 0	8 12
31	9 6		9 1	

If you like, this information can be shown in a frequency table (Table 3). It is also possible to plot weight for any month on a graph: Fig. 1 shows the daily weights for our hypothetical slimmer in January.

Table 3 Frequency table for the information given in Table 2

Weight	Number of days at given weight			
st lb	January	February	March	April
9 8	8	0	0	0
9 7	12	5	0	0
9 6	5	5	0	0
9 5	5	6	0	0
9 4	1	6	3	0
9 3	0	5	11	1
9 2	0	1	8	3
9 1	0	0	5	9
9 0	0	0	4	9
8 13	0	0	0	4
8 12	0	0	0	3
8 11	0	0	0	1

If your graphs and charts are showing an overall decrease in weight, then you know you are eating the right amounts. However, if you feel progress is too slow, you need to make slight adjustments to your food and exercise programme to get it going as you want it. You are not looking for a fast drop in weight. You want a relatively slow but controlled and permanent solution to your weight problem. The methods we have outlined will ensure that your will-power is strong enough for you to attain your goals.

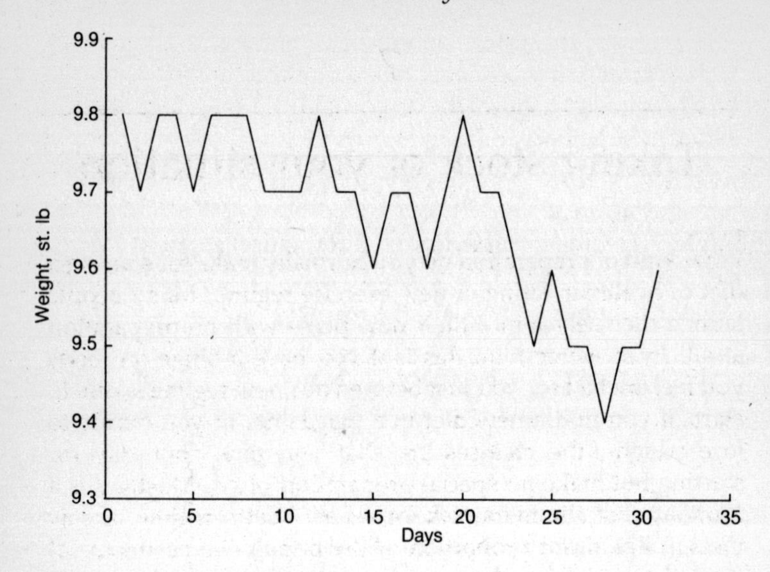

Fig. 1. Graph showing daily weight record for the hypothetical slimmer in January.

7

Taking stock of your situation

What kind of preparation do you normally make for starting a diet or healthier eating or new exercise regime? Many people launch themselves into their new plans with no preparation at all. Even worse than this is if you have a binge on foods you feel are bad for you just before your new regime is due to start. If you find a new diet in a magazine, or you decide to lose weight, the chances are that you pick your day for starting but make no special preparation plans. Mostly it is a Monday that slimmers pick for a new health regime, a new diet. A significant proportion of the population seems to eat less on Mondays; not so many are on their new diet by the time Sunday comes around. Diets started without preparation are broken all too easily. If you do not have enough of the right kinds of food, or if you have too many high-fat, high-sugar foods in the cupboard, it is difficult to keep strictly to a diet.

We strongly recommend that you spend a week, or preferably two, preparing for your new regime. You need to take stock of your situation properly and plan the course of action most likely to work for you. You need to find what is right with your current life-style, in terms of food and exercise, and what needs improvement. You need to establish a list of goals and decide when and in what order you will introduce change to your eating habits. You have to buy a diary, graph paper and, possibly, weighing scales. You should get someone to sponsor you, and organize your own system of rewards. Your weekly shopping list will probably change; you need to think about the best ways to do this for you. Some new exercise clothes might be a good idea if you can afford it, and you might like to investigate local exercise groups or sports clubs. A set of 'before' photos need to be taken. Clearly you are not going to do all this in an hour, in an afternoon, or even in a day or two. You are about to set out on an interesting and formative experience, something that is likely to have a major impact on your life. A week or two spent in preparation is really a comparatively short time to plan the necessary changes.

Step 1: buy the essential things for recording progress

The first thing to do is go on a shopping trip. You will need to buy a reasonably large diary. It is highly unlikely that you will be doing this around January but diaries are available from many stores at most times of the year. The pages that contain dates already past can be divided into sections, such as 'favourite recipes'; 'goals for weight', 'food change, and exercise'; 'lists of rewards'; 'weight charts'. If you cannot find a diary, buy a large notebook instead.

Some diaries contain sheets of paper printed as graph paper. If your diary or notebook does not have these, or does not contain enough of them for your needs, buy a small packet of graph paper as well. Should you be lucky enough to own a 'Filofax', there are many kinds of graph paper, different coloured notepapers, and diary sheets that you can purchase to make into a comprehensive section on your new diet and health programme.

In addition to all this, now is the time to buy your new weighing scales. Also, on this first shopping trip, purchase a film for your camera and a large photograph album where you can keep a record of your progress in picture form. Finally, look in a large magazine shop for a booklet guide to calorie values. Some slimming magazines also publish guides to the fat and fibre content of food. These guides are not absolutely essential (the outline on nutrition in Chapter 4 tells you all you really need to know about healthy eating), but they can be very interesting; the better ones give information about foods under specific brand names. Some large chains of supermarkets publish booklets on calorie, fat, and fibre content of their foods. If none of this additional information interests you, an excellent alternative is to read the labels on the foods you already buy to find their content and nutrition value.

If you have bought a booklet on calorie values (or fats or fibres) pick a typical day's eating during this preparation phase and work out the total value for that day. Think about how the result could be most easily improved.

You do not need to start changing your health-related habits until this preparation phase of one or two weeks is complete. During the whole of this phase eat and exercise exactly as you normally do. Do *not* try to give yourself a head start by dieting earlier than you should. Do not binge. You should not feel any pressure to eat all your favourite things before your diet begins because when you do start, food change will be so gradual that you will notice no hardship. You will still be eating the foods you enjoy. Therefore if during this first shopping trip of your preparation phase you want to pop in somewhere for a drink and a snack (assuming that this is fairly usual for you), go ahead and do it. Throughout the preparation days you will be establishing a baseline record of your eating and exercise behaviour as it normally occurs.

Step 2: review the contents of your food cupboards

A good start to identifying and describing your normal eating habits is to write a list of the contents of your food cupboards and fridge. Make a note of this somewhere near the beginning of your diary. Do not buy in any special food or drink or alter anything from what is usually there. Leave a page next to this one in your diary where you will be able to record the contents of your cupboard at the end of your diet when all your goals have been reached. The basics of good nutrition lie in what is readily available in your house for you to consume. Should you have food in other places besides the kitchen, record this too. Put each item on a separate line in the diary. Here is an example:

Fridge:	Six eggs, two bottles of silver top milk, Cheddar cheese, one pack of lard, one pack of butter.
Freezer:	Pack of steaks, beefburgers, fish-fingers, peas, runner beans, ready cooked curry meal, cod.
Cupboard:	Two tins of baked beans, part pack of biscuits, three tins of peas, box muesli, two bags of sugar, white rice, two bars of chocolate, one sponge cake, white spaghetti.
Vegetable rack:	Potatoes, carrots, onions.
Living room:	Two apples.
Pocket:	Part pack of mints.

This is probably nowhere near as long as your list but it gives you some idea of how much detail is needed in recording items. It is easiest to list foods and drinks according to the location in which they are stored.

The next step is to take a pen and put a tick against any item that you feel is absolutely fine, could not be improved upon and should continue as a major part of any healthy diet. Go back to Chapter 4 to remind yourself of some of the basics of good nutrition if you need to. Out of all the items in our list we would probably tick the apples, potatoes, carrots, onions, cod and the frozen peas and beans. Now, many of the other items are also sound and have a part to play but they could be improved upon. For example, the silver top milk could be replaced by skimmed or semi-skimmed milk; a cooking fat is alright, but replace the lard with sunflower oil; the muesli probably contains added sugar and a sugar-free brand would be better; the rice and spaghetti could both be brown instead of white. Some of the items are fine as they are but are not given unconditional approval because they should only be eaten in moderation. So, items like eggs and cheese are fine but to have, say, a three-egg omelette with three or four ounces (113 g) of cheese added would be far too fatty a meal with no fibre. Looking at your own list of food you can write comments and suggestions for improvement next to each item. Finally, there are clearly a number of items on our food list that are relatively low in nutritional value and high in saturated fat and/or sugar. Put a cross against these. From our list we would choose to put a cross against sugar, chocolate, biscuits, sponge cake, and mints. This is not to say that you should never eat these things but that ultimately they should play a minimal part in your day-to-day eating. Next to each item with a cross on your list write some alternatives for you to try. For example, you might choose to bake a low-sugar sponge cake. Some brands of biscuits are made with wholemeal flour or oats and slightly less sugar, which might be some improvement on your usual brand. Even if you do not want to change brands you can decide to eat fewer biscuits or have something else like fresh fruit instead. Write such suggestions on the line next to the relevant item. These are our comments on just some of the things on our list. These examples should give you some idea of how to approach your own list of foods. Go through your whole list with a critical eye. For some items it might be difficult to decide whether to use approval or put a cross against an item. For some things you may find it difficult to see how to improve on them or you will not be able to think of suitable substitutes. Just make the best decision you possibly can in the light of the information contained in Chapter 4. This will serve to start you in a new way of thinking about your eating habits.

Step 3: shopping for food

During this preparation phase we do not want you to change your shopping habits when buying food. However, next time you go to a large supermarket for your supplies (or if you shop daily, the next time you go to your local shops) consider your buying habits. Do you always go for the same kinds of things? Which shelves do you rush past? Are there healthier, low-fat, low-sugar foods or drinks available that you do not usually notice? Just make a mental note of what is around.

Consider, too, how you normally shop. Fairly typical for a week is one main shop at a supermarket plus buying in the odd thing during the week. Are these the best options for you? Is there a good fresh fish market near by? How often do you go to it? Could you buy in quite a bit of fresh fish, say ten portions if you plan to have ten fish meals in a month, so that there is always good healthy protein food available as a base for a meal? Have you ever been around a health-food shop? Try it and see if anything there appeals to you. If you live a fast, hectic life and you eat mostly ready-made convenience foods, try to consider some other alternatives. For example, you could make batches of meals from fresh food, then freeze them. If you own a microwave oven, jacket potatoes take very little time to cook yet form a base for a tasty meal (add tuna, beans, sweetcorn, cottage cheese or whatever low-fat filling takes your fancy). At this stage simply consider what you normally do but also review the other options that are open to you. For a new system to work it needs to be flexible and to fit in with your own personal requirements.

Step 4: start using your diary to record your daily food-intake, exercise, and weight

What you need is a record of seven to ten days of fairly typical intake of food and drink. Once you have your diary you will probably be able to start this straight away. Do not try to perfect your normal eating routine. Just write it all as it happens. If the seven- to ten-day period includes the odd party or meal out (and this is something you occasionally do) just record all the details. Do not abstain.

The only reason for not beginning your diary straight away is if the next seven to ten days covers a really unusual time, for example your annual holiday, or a bout of sickness, or Christmas and New Year. Otherwise you can begin. If you are a person who usually eats roughly the same amounts each day, with regular meal times, a typical pattern will quickly reveal itself in the diary; keep it for only seven days. However, if your eating habits are fairly erratic and you eat far less or very differently on some days than on others, keep the diary for ten days (or longer if necessary) until a picture of your eating habits emerges.

Each day that you record your food intake make sure to make a fairly detailed account. You will not be making such time-consuming notes after this preparation phase, so bear with it. You need to have detailed information to help you plan your goals for healthier eating and weight control.

Table 4 is an example of a typical day's food intake. You can see the kind of detail you need to record. (In fact, if you want to work out calories on the odd day you will need to have even more detail than this: you will need to weigh out quantities of food, including things like butter, you should note the make of chocolate biscuit, and so on.) However, for our purposes the kind of detail in our example should be sufficient. You must note down if there is added sugar or salt or fat in food or drink, as well as the type of food or drink you are having. Note, too, if food is tinned, fresh, or frozen.

When you come to make your list of goals you will be able to spot themes and trends from your diary records. You can look at your eating habits and consider easy places to start change. The details of this will be explained fully in the next chapter.

Go through your seven- to ten-day diary and compare what you actually eat with the kinds of food we recommend in Chapter 4. Consider what you could eat more of, as well as what you should cut down on. Could your consumption of fresh fruit and vegetables be increased? Are you getting enough of good carbohydrate foods like bread, pasta, and rice? How many meals contain low-fat protein like chicken and fish? Could these be used to replace some other fattier

Table 4 Daily food intake before dieting

Day/date	Time	Place	Food consumed
Monday	08.00	Bed	Coffee with silver top milk and one spoon of sugar, one chocolate biscuit.
	08.45	Kitchen	One slice of white toast spread with generous portion of salted butter, two teaspoons of marmalade, coffee with silver top milk and one spoon of sugar.
	12.45	Kitchen	Fish and chips, orange squash.
	15.00	Lounge	Coffee with silver top milk and one spoon of sugar, two chocolate biscuits.
	18.00	Kitchen	Potato mashed with generous portion of salted butter, more salt, and a dash of silver top milk; grilled pork chop and tinned peas; apple; coffee with silver top milk and one teaspoon of sugar.
	21.00	Lounge	Packet of crisps.
	22.00	Lounge	Cup of hot chocolate made with silver top milk and one spoon of sugar.

meals a few times a week? Use a green pencil to underline all the foods or meals you normally eat that you think are nutritionally sound and that you do not want to change. Use a red pencil to underline the things you think are not so good for you and should be restricted. Use an orange or yellow pencil for the remainder, that is, things you are unsure about or which do not seem to fit clearly into either the good or the bad categories.

As well as food and drink, get into the habit of recording your weight each day. This does not take much time and it will be something that you will continue after this preparation phase is over.

Finally, record the exercise that you take on each day that you record the details of your food and drink. Obviously you will have to use some initiative here in deciding what constitutes recordable exercise. A game of tennis, a jog, a swim, a weight-lifting session, or a yoga session are all obvious examples of exercise to record. If you do not do anything like this, but on the other hand you do walk a fair amount each day (to the shops, to work, etc.) record either the distance or the time spent in walking each day. Do not, however, record every time you put one foot in front of the other. Going up one flight of stairs to visit the lavatory is not worth recording as exercise for the average person!

Be as active as you normally are. When you analyse your exercise levels at the end of the preparation phase consider the amount you do. Do you ever become breathless because you are having a really good work out? Does anything you do sustain a slightly increased heart-rate for 20 to 30 minutes? Of all your exercise, which enhances stamina, which is for suppleness, and which for strength? Are you lacking anywhere?

Step 5: final preparation

When your seven- to ten-day recording has finished you should be ready to list your goals for change. Just before we show you how to do this, check some final details. Are your 'before' photographs taken? Have you checked out the local sports facilities? If you have made up your mind what you are going to do, go shopping for necessary extras like jogging shoes, or walking shoes, or a swimming costume. Prepare a section in your diary for recipes; in future you will not be recording everything you eat but you need to start your own personal tried and tested recipe book. Check over all the things you have written down earlier in the preparation phase and make sure you have a full picture of yourself as regards health-related habits.

You can see that the preparation is long and complex, but now it is virtually over. It will enable you to decide upon a list of goals for weight change, exercise, and food change. Only when this is done will you be properly ready to embark on your new health regime.

8

How to make your list of goals

Goal-setting starts with a good analytical look through your diary. Do not regard your record of baseline behaviour, your seven- to ten-day preparation phase, with an overly pessimistic, critical eye. Use your diary to form a picture of the kind of person you are when it comes to food intake. What are your preferences? For example, do you find you eat once, twice, three times a day? Alternatively, are you a 'nibbler', consuming food ten times a day or more? Is there a certain time when you always love to sit down with a relaxing drink and something to eat? Is your supper drink or your afternoon cup of tea a sacred ritual for you? Basically, decide on your preferences here. You need to adapt any healthy diet to your own individual style of life; you need to be able to live the way you want to. Make a mental note of the things you find are most important to you and also of the things you habitually do that could perhaps go without too much hardship because they are not an essential part of your well-being and happiness.

Right from the very start it will help if you can decide at least on the number of main meals you will have each day and on the number of snacks, if any. Fix these in your mind as units you will have to work on to make each of them as nutritionally sound as possible. Do not eat mindlessly, do not eat unless you are properly hungry, and do not be afraid to leave food once you are full. Think about any new routines you wish to establish from the beginning, such as a day for a new recipe each week, new shopping routines, different meal times, or restricted locations to keep food in the house.

You are now ready to set your goals for change. No two people's set of goals will be the same. The decisions you make concerning the right goals for you will depend on your current weight, your optimum weight, and the eating and exercise habits you recorded in your preparation phase. What we offer here is a guide for you to follow when you list your own goals. The example we shall give is for a person who starts the regime moderately overweight and whose normal meals are fairly typically too high in fat, sugar, and salt, and too low in fibre. This hypothetical person (in this case, female) also has done very little sport or exercise for years.

To give you a more complete picture, this individual is 30 lb (13.6 kg) overweight (has dieted on and off but tends to end up back at square one). She takes little exercise, does not even walk much, and prefers to use the car or public transport. She would not do very well on any test of strength, stamina, or suppleness. She normally eats three meals a day but sometimes misses breakfast. She usually has a snack mid-morning, at around 4 pm, and later in the evening while watching television.

When breakfast is taken it usually consists of cereal and milk, or toast spread with hard margarine or butter and jam or marmalade. Milk with this meal (and with all drinks throughout the day) is silver top full-fat. Breakfast cereals are mostly sugar-coated; when she occasionally has a wholegrain cereal (like Weetabix) she adds two teaspoons of sugar. All hot drinks also each have two teaspoons of sugar added.

Lunch is often a sandwich or something on toast (like cheese or eggs) or a pie or pasty. Bread is usually white, although she buys wholegrain brown bread occasionally. Butter or hard margarine is always spread lavishly on bread. Sometimes a piece of fruit or a tub of yogurt is eaten at the end of lunch but more often she finishes with a biscuit or has nothing as dessert.

The evening meal might be potatoes, meat or fish, and vegetables. All fresh and frozen vegetables are cooked with salt. Salt and butter or hard margarine also added to vegetables after cooking. Meat products often include pastry or are fairly fatty (like sausages or chops). Vegetables may be fresh, frozen, or tinned. Occasionally pasta or rice is used as a base for a meal rather than potatoes. Both are white rather than wholegrain and both are cooked with salt. Fast evening meals would be, for example: cheese omelette; egg and chips; and pizza or complete convenience meal cooked from frozen; pie and chips (take-away). Dessert is usually something like a biscuit or small piece of cake or rice pudding or pie and custard (but dessert is not eaten every night).

Snacks through the day are usually sweet (such as a small bar of chocolate or a piece of cake or a biscuit). Snacks in the evening are more often savoury (such as salted nuts or crisps).

Now, your diary may reveal a picture like this in some respects, or your eating habits may be totally different. Either way, when you see how we establish lists of goals for this person you can learn some simple principles for establishing your own goals.

Notice the time element, that is just how slowly this person is expected to change. Especially in the early weeks of the diet, eating habits are very similar to the old ways. Our dieter is not launched into a totally unrealistic programme. Yet at the end of one year all the health-related goals are attained and she has attained her correct weight. Even if you personally have much more of a weight problem than this dieter, do not try to speed up change too much. A loss of 2–3 lb (around 1 kg) per month totals about 30 lb (13.6 kg) in a year, 60 lb (27. 2kg) in two years, and a huge 90 lb or 6 st 6 lb (40.8kg) in three years! Go slowly, go carefully, and enjoy the process of change. Your lists of goals should not put undue pressure on you; you should not feel stressed. Rather, your list of goals should act as signposts to a pleasurable trip.

Goals for weight change

You will be faced here with a great temptation to set goals for fast weight loss that will prove difficult or impossible for you to achieve. Ideally it would be nice to be the perfect shape tomorrow or next week, but this just is not going to happen. The woman we have just described is 30 lb (13.6 kg) overweight and she should be delighted if she can be rid of this in around a year.

Imagine friends that you see only once a year, say at Christmas time. If one of your friends lost this amount of weight from one Christmas to the next, changed from a fat person into a slim and healthy person, you would certainly notice! Now, 30 lb in a year is a loss of between 2 and 3 lb (about 1 kg) a month. The dieter in our example therefore wants to think in terms of an average loss of a mere half a pound (a quarter of a kilogram) each week. This is actually 26 lb (11.8 kg) of fat in a year. If she loses this gigantic amount in a year she should be happy. She also wants to exercise to improve muscle tone during this period; she can then see what shape she is in at the end of the year before she decides whether or not she really does need to lose those extra 4 lb (1.8 kg).

We have already stressed at the end of Chapter 6 how important it is to record your daily weight and also to chart it and plot it on a monthly graph. At this stage, while setting your goals for the whole dieting period, use another graph to plot out your weight at the end of each month. This one sheet of graph paper for our dieter will therefore have twelve points marked on it along the bottom axis (one for each month) and around thirty points marked on the other axis (each point representing 1 lb or 0.45 kg). She can then mark faintly in pencil an 'aim' line. She can pencil in the weight she hopes to be at the end of each month. The actual weight at the end of each month can then be filled in as the weight control regime progresses. Although change in weight is very noticeable after a few months or a year, it simply is not detectable by just looking at physical shape on a daily basis. Graphs and charts are really important as a means of providing a simple, clear guide to progress.

As a final point on goal-setting for weight, there is nothing wrong with being slightly under or over your goal weight for any one day or week. However, do not try to be too far away from it. Do not deliberately aim to go greatly below it. You may occasionally find you drop quite a bit of weight fairly suddenly. For example, some people find this when they start on their goals for salt reduction (they lose excess water). Or you may find that when you first start on your weight control programme you lose the first 3–5 lb (1.4–2.3 kg) fairly rapidly. This is fine. If you go about this amount below your 'aim' line on your graph do not be too concerned. Consider it as a kind of insurance for the odd times when you are not losing weight quite as you should. Ideally, you should adjust your eating so that you are meeting your aims for goal weights or are at least 2 to 3 lb (1 kg) within your goal weight for any particular week.

Goals for food change: sugar, fat, fibre, and salt

Goals for sugar reduction

Look at your diary of the seven to ten days of recorded eating and decide on the major sources of sugar present. Our hypothetical dieter described earlier has plenty of sugar. She takes two teaspoons of sugar in each of her hot drinks; she adds two teaspoons of sugar to her breakfast cereal (or has sugar-coated cereal or muesli with sugar). If she has toast she spreads it with jam or marmalade. She often eats biscuits or some kind of sweet dessert after each of her two main meals of the day. Snacks in the day are also usually sweet (biscuit, cake, or chocolate). She is a nibbler. She is not keen to eliminate all these sources of sugar because she derives such pleasure from them. However, she has decided to give herself a year to change. Here is her list of sugar goals. Each goal should last one week before she moves on to add the next goal to her eating behaviour. She has graded these goals in terms of difficulty; she starts with the easiest things first. You should use this strategy too; make sure you start with the simplest changes for you.

Sugar at breakfast:

1. Reduce sugar on cereal to one and a half teaspoons.
2. Reduce sugar on cereal to one teaspoon.
3. Try a reduced-sugar jam on the toast.
4. Buy cereals that are not sugar-coated and sugar-free museli.

Sugar at lunch:

5. No more than one biscuit or two squares of chocolate at the end of lunch.
6. Fresh fruit (instead of biscuit or two squares of chocolate) at the end of lunch on two days a week.
7. Fresh fruit after lunch on a third day each week.
8. Fresh fruit after lunch on a fourth day each week.
9. Fresh fruit after lunch five days each week. (This still leaves two days where lunch can be finished by either a biscuit or two squares of chocolate.)

Sugar at the evening meal:

10. Decrease the size of the sweet dessert to about three-quarters of the usual amount.
11. Decrease the portion of dessert to about half the usual amount.
12. Look up recipes for no-sugar or low-sugar desserts and try out one or two.
13. Have fresh fruit or sugar-free yogurt for dessert on one day a week.
14. Have the fruit or yogurt for dessert on a second day each week.
15. Try some more low-sugar or no-sugar dessert recipes.
16. Have fresh fruit or sugar-free yogurt for dessert a minimum of three days a week; the other days have low-

sugar or no-sugar dessert recipes whenever possible (e.g. unless eating out or at a friend's house).

Sugar in drinks:

17. Reduce to one-and-a-half spoons of sugar per cup.
18. Reduce to just one spoon per cup.
19. Only half a spoon of sugar per cup.
20. Remain on the goal for Week 19 for a bit longer to get used to the less sweet taste.
21. No sugar in cups of coffee or other warm beverages.
22. All cold ready-made drinks (like squash or cola) to be the no-sugar kind (buy either the so-called diet low-calorie drinks or mineral water like Perrier); freshly squeezed fruit juice is quite acceptable (free of refined sugar).

Sweet snacks in the day:

23. Restrict the number of snacks on sugary items (the odd sweet or biscuit; chocolate; cake) to five times per day.
24. Restrict sugary snacks to four times per day.
25. Reduce sugary snacks to three times a day.
26. Reduce sugary snacks to twice a day. One snack should constitute, at most, half a bar of chocolate, or two biscuits or a very small cake (or anything sweet of around 100–150 calories). These sweet snacks do not *have* to be eaten each day (savoury snacks or fruit would be much better).

These twenty-six goals should take twenty-six weeks to complete. Therefore after six months the dieter is behaving according to all twenty-six goals and she has achieved a considerable reduction in sugar intake. All the little steps have added up to a high achievement. She still, of course, has some sugar. If, like her, you have a sweet tooth, you might be better leaving just a little sugar in the diet to increase the likelihood that you will continue with the new sugar-reduced regime. Our dieter still has another six months to go until all her weight goals have been achieved. As she will be maintaining all her twenty-six goals on a permanent basis, the low sugar intake should help her considerably in getting down to her final goal weight for the end of the year.

Goals for reduction of saturated fat

Each week, as well as the weight goal and the sugar goal, there will be a separate goal for the reduction of saturated fat. Our dieter derives large quantities of saturated fat from a number of sources: full-fat dairy products such as silver top milk, cheddar and other hard cheese; eggs; butter, hard margarine, lard and blended vegetable oils; meats such as beef, pork, lamb; meat products like sausages, pies and burgers; crisps and nuts; chocolate, cake, biscuits, and ice-cream. These last four items also contain sugar and have already appeared in the list of goals for sugar reduction. They therefore need not appear here as well.

The principles for establishing lists of goals for fat reduction are similar to those for sugar reduction, namely, do the things that are easiest first; use lots of small, easy steps; spend about a week trying to behave according to that week's goal (and with all preceding ones being maintained) before going on to add the next goal to your repertoire. Again, your own lists of goals will depend on your areas of strengths and weaknesses and on your own preference for the order in which to tackle things. Here is the list of fat goals for our hypothetical dieter.

Reducing fat from meat:

1. Cut visible fat off meat.
2. Use slightly less meat (less by about one third) when making up meals like chilli con carne or stews. Add more vegetables instead.
3. Leave some of the pastry crust when having meat pies.
4. Have poultry once or twice a week.

5. As well as poultry once or twice, also have fish at least twice a week.
6. Buy low-fat sausages to replace the standard ones and have fewer sausages in the meal.

Reducing saturated fat from spreads and oils:

7. Remove a small quantity of butter from the fridge so that it softens and is easier to spread, then spread it very thinly on bread.
8. Use about half the usual quantity of butter or hard margarine on vegetables.
9. Stop using butter on vegetables; experiment with different herbs instead.
10. Use polyunsaturated margarine instead of butter on most occasions.
11. Grill rather than fry foods whenever possible.
12. Reduce the amount of fat in recipes by at least one quarter.
13. Have chips no more than twice a week and if preparing them at home have them cut very thick.
14. Use sunflower oil or safflower oil instead of lard or blended vegetable oils.

Reducing saturated fat from dairy products:

15. Buy semi-skimmed milk to replace silver top milk.
16. Have cream a maximum of once a week.
17. Have less hard cheese; use it grated rather than having slabs of it.
18. Use skimmed-milk instead of semi-skimmed.

Reducing fat from savoury snacks like crisps and nuts:

19. Have either one packet of crisps or a measured 1 oz. of nuts each day.

20. One packet of crisps or 1 oz. of nuts on six days in the week.
21. One packet of crisps or 1 oz. of nuts on five days in the week.
22. One packet of crisps or 1 oz. of nuts on four days in the week.
23. One packet of crisps or 1 oz. of nuts on three days in the week.

It should take 23 weeks for all 23 goals to be accomplished. You can see that there need not be the same number of fat goals as sugar goals. Just use as many goals as are necessary for you.

Reducing salt

Salt is present in many foods. Most people have far too much salt and would do well to reduce salt from major sources such as: salt added in cooking and at table; tinned vegetables and some convenience meals (read labels); tinned and packet soups, many sauces and gravies; salted meats such as bacon; salted fish. Some take-away foods (such as Chinese meals) often contain large quantities of salt. If you become very thirsty after such a meal this is a sign of high salt content. Some snacks like crisps and some nuts also have obvious added salt. However, as these foods also contain fat they have already been incorporated under the goals for fat and so need not be repeated here.

What follows is the list of goals for salt reduction for our typical dieter. You might find, like her, that it can be difficult to divide up salt reduction into many small steps. What she has chosen to do, therefore, is to have only ten goals, but to spend two weeks on each goal.

Goals for salt

1. Salted meat or salted fish only three times a week maximum.

2. Salted meat or salted fish only twice a week maximum.
3. Home-made salt-free soup recipes instead of tinned or packet soups.
4. Stop using salt when cooking rice or pasta.
5. Use three-quarters the usual amount of salt when cooking vegetables.
6. Use half the usual amount of salt when cooking vegetables.
7. Use one quarter the usual amount of salt when cooking vegetables.
8. Buy a low-sodium table salt (or a potassium salt).
9. Use no salt in cooking vegetables.
10. Use no salt when cooking any food at all.

After twenty weeks this dieter will have attained all the salt goals. If you find that your taste for salt is slow to disappear, there is no reason why you should not spend three or even four weeks on each goal. If our dieter had done this she would still have achieved what she set out to achieve within her dieting year.

Increasing fibre

The final list of goals for food change is obviously rather different from all the others because the aim is to increase consumption of something rather than decrease it. Also you may well find that you enjoy a variety of fibre-rich foods and it is no hardship to increase your intake relatively quickly. The feeling of fullness you acquire from, say, jacket potato or brown rice or wholemeal bread can certainly help compensate for the restriction of saturated fat and refined sugar. There are only seven goals in our dieter's list to achieve a considerable and beneficial increase in fibre. You can have a much longer list if you feel you require it, or spend a few weeks on each goal before adding another goal.

Goals for fibre:

1 .Have pulses (peas or beans) with one meal each day (for example, a portion of peas to accompany fish or meat; red beans in chilli; peas or lentils added to a curry; beans on toast; lentil soup; a corn on the cob).
2. At least one piece of fresh fruit each day (preferably two or three).
3. Other vegetables or salad at least once each day.
4. Breakfast cereal to be wholegrain.
5. All bread to be wholegrain.
6. Rice to be wholegrain.
7. Pasta to be 'whole' too.

Goals for exercise

Your own goals will be determined by your current level of exercise, your current fitness. We shall give you a list for our typical inactive person with a weight problem. Each goal is planned for a week but some may possibly require longer; our dieter will have to take extra time if it is taking her body longer to adjust than she anticipates at the start. The goals cover exercise for stamina, strength, and suppleness. If necessary go back to Chapter 5 to remind yourself of appropriate forms of exercise to cover these three areas (choose the things you like the best to get you fit).

Goals for exercise

1. walk briskly for ten minutes each day.
2. Walk briskly for twenty minutes each day.
3. Walk briskly for thirty minutes each day.
4. Buy an exercise tape (or video) that covers general aerobics (exercises for suppleness and strength, plus stamina if they are done fast enough). Do these once each week (with a thirty-minute walk on the six other days).

5. Aerobics Mondays and Fridays; a thirty-minute walk on the other five days.
6. Join an evening yoga class (once a week); do aerobics once or twice a week, plus a thirty-minute walk three times a week.

It is fine to stay at this kind of level for a while. Once the dieter starts to lose weight and feels more energetic it might be time to consider further possibilities. For example, when the course of yoga finishes an advanced class might be available. A different sport might be incorporated occasionally. Brisk walking might progress to jogging. It can be fun to be flexible in your approach to physical exercise. As your fitness increases you should find that you are naturally walking places rather than going by bus or car. You should move more quickly, bounding up stairs and so on. You might not need, therefore, to deliberately incorporate a walk as a daily goal as it will be happening anyway. This will leave you free to concentrate on having other more specific exercise or sports sessions as goals. As we mentioned in Chapter 5, at this stage you need only time-table three or perhaps four exercise routines per week (where you get slightly breathless at each session for a half-hour period) in order to keep up a reasonable degree of fitness.

At last you are ready to get properly started on your own personal health and fitness programme. You have spent a while analysing your typical eating and exercise habits. You have a much greater understanding of your own behaviour patterns and the things that motivate you, and this has helped you established your own list of goals. These easy steps to well-being should be fun to achieve. Each one should have its own reward and, of course, the ultimate reward of a new, slimmer, fitter you will gradually develop over the course of the weight reduction programme.

9

Keeping to your programme until all your goals are achieved

Once you have all your lists of goals written somewhere at the front of your diary, you are ready to start. What do you actually record in your diary week by week? There is no need at all to write down all your food and drink each day, although you can do this occasionally if you find it motivates you. What you must do, however, is to write down your weekly goals at the beginning of each week. Just do this as you go along. For example, for the typical dieter we described in the last chapter, her goals for Week 1 are as follows.

Goal for weight change To lose half a pound (0.25 kg) of fat. In practice it is difficult to accurately measure such a small drop, and weight does fluctuate a little anyway from day to day. She therefore would like to see at least two or three days where her weight drops below her starting weight, maybe by 1 lb (0.5 kg). She obviously does not want to go above her starting weight if she can help it. (The following week the goal is again to lose half a pound of fat (0.25 kg), so she would hope on Week 2 to be below her starting weight by at least 1 lb (0.5 kg) on most days).

Goal for sugar Reduce sugar on cereal to one and a half spoonsful.

Goal for fat Cut visible fat off meat in meat meals.

Goal for salt Salted meat or salted fish only three times a week in total.

Goal for fibre Have pulses with one meal each day.

Goal for exercise Walk briskly for ten minutes each day.

The rewards for the end of the week should also be written in the diary in the space for Week 1. This is all she has to do at the beginning of the week. She should record her daily weight. She could also write down if she has any problems with any of these goals, or any spectacular successes (like a new recipe or a new idea for places to shop for food). She can note down details of any situation she has difficulty coping with, and just what strategies she used to try to overcome problematic situations. She should also write down anything about which she feels particularly proud, such as doing well with some new exercise.

Eating during the first week will be very similar to that on baseline days during the preparation phase (because only the first goals in the lists will be introduced). Nevertheless, quantities of food will need to be adjusted in order to achieve the desired weight goals. Right from the beginning the dieter should be learning to eat according to internal hunger cues and not to binge. If the dieter feels she needs extra guidance or added structure to meal planning, she can always refer back to the suggested meals for good nutrition that we gave at the end of Chapter 4. It is necessary for you to take this kind of positive approach; think in terms of maximizing the number of nutrients that you derive from food by eating the right kind of balance of different foods during meals.

During the second week our dieter will move on to her next set of goals. She should now aim to be 1 lb (0.5 kg) below her starting weight on most days; she should reduce sugar on cereal to just one teaspoon; she should use less meat when making up meat meals like stews, using more vegetables instead (this is as well, of course, as maintaining the goal for fat reduction from Week 1); she should have salted meat or salted fish only three times a week in total (you will remember that salt goals last for two weeks each); she should have one or two pieces of fresh fruit each day (this is as well as the goal for Week 1, having pulses with one meal each day); she should have a brisk twenty-minute walk each day.

You should continue the goal-achieving process in the same way as our example dieter. Eventually all your goals will be achieved and all your rewards earned. Occasionally there will be additional problems. For example, you may have to make special provision for Christmas week or holidays. Do not just give yourself the whole week off. Write down the goals for the week as usual. Then allocate 'free periods' when meals can be eaten exactly as you wish, for example over Christmas you could have one 'free' meal each day for three or four days. You might have to allow yourself more than this if you are away from home and someone else is preparing food for you. However, continue to weigh each day if at all possible. Do not over-eat. Eat what is on offer and enjoy it without guilt, but stop when you have had enough. If you know that a dessert is likely to be particularly rich but it is something you relish, then do not eat so much of the main course; you will then be hungry enough to enjoy the dessert without feeling sick or bloated. Should you find that despite all this you do occasionally eat too much, try to take extra exercise, the occasional long walk at least, to work it off.

If things go wrong

Every now and again you will not make the progress that you anticipate. Things can sometimes go wrong suddenly. For example, you are lucky enough to have a holiday abroad for two or three weeks but you have no access to scales and you also eat out all the time. When you arrive back you weigh 7 lb (about 3 kg) more than you did when you went away. You look like you have blown up like a balloon and you feel that you are a complete dieting failure. As a consequence of this you are tempted to either stop your regime entirely and remain fat, or start a crash diet. Do not do either of these things. A crash diet will leave you hungry, you will binge and you will not get anywhere. Do not abandon your programme either. However, you will need to decide just where to restart it. A good place to begin is with the goals that you had reached about two weeks before you went on holiday. There is no need to go back to square one; just a few steps backward is all that is needed. Many people find that the weight drops off quickly once the holiday has finished. The chances are that your holiday food was somewhat higher in salt than the diet to which you have become accustomed so you might be retaining 2–3 lb (1 kg) of excess water. Also there is a high probability that your holiday meals were lower in roughage than your own regime at home. Therefore you might also be constipated and heavier because your intestines are holding extra food. So there is no need for despair. A couple of weeks should see you safely back on your way to successful weight control.

Your programme might also suddenly go wrong for no obvious external reason. You might just get to a goal that is difficult to master, or you could find that when you are about half-way through your goals you get stuck and can go no further. There are a number of strategies at your disposal and you can use one or a mixture of them to help you over an unexpected hurdle. First, if you find a goal difficult to achieve, you might bypass it, put the goal later on the list. Alternatively, you might break the goal down into smaller mini-goals, and spread these over a few weeks. This obviously gives you longer to adapt to the necessary changes. It could well be, also, that you were over-optimistic when you made your original lists. Yet another strategy is to put progress on 'hold' and stay with your current level of progress for a few weeks until you feel more accustomed to the level and better able to proceed.

Instead of finding sudden problems you might find that progress slowly grinds to a halt. You find that you do not always keep to your goals. You have the occasional binge. Perhaps you even regain some weight. Whatever goes wrong, do not try to punish yourself or start feeling guilty, because then you will tend to seek out food as a comfort. This is what you do not want to happen! Instead you should investigate the reasons why progress has faltered by taking an analytical look through your diary. You should have noted down successes and also failures. What is it about any situation that stops you succeeding? Are you too hungry and vulnerable at any particular time? Should your goals be made smaller and then into a longer list? Does your meal planning need more structure? Is a certain situation or a certain person tempting you to eat the things you do not really want? What can you do to change this? Is the reward level high enough?

Never blame yourself for anything that goes wrong. Life does not always go to plan. It is difficult for you to foresee at the beginning of your programme just how you will feel, what things will happen, which goals might prove harder than anticipated. You will find out about these things as time goes on. Experience will show you how to readjust your programme to get yourself back on the right track. You have time on your side.

When things go well

If your preparation phase and goal setting has been done carefully and you do not expect yourself to do too much too soon, you should find that for the most part you succeed. You should find yourself working slowly and carefully through your goal lists. Do not try to speed up progress by doing more goals in any one week than you should. This is likely to lead to undue pressure on you and you will start to break from the programme and put on weight.

You will need time to adjust to your new body image. Enjoy the process of change. Other people will also have to adjust to the new you. It may be tempting to talk a great deal about what you have learned about diet, nutrition, exercise, and weight control. Do not be over-enthusiastic and bore people. There are other things going on in life. Keep the business of weight control in perspective.

Epilogue

Let us assume that within a certain time, probably around a year or so for most people, you will have achieved your ideal weight, a good, firm shape, and a reasonable level of physical fitness. Is it now time to throw away the charts and graphs, have a ceremonial burning of the diary? In brief, no, it is not. The period of time just after you have attained all your goals is something of a danger period; this is when many dieters lapse back into their old ways. You, of course, have many advantages over the average dieter. Your own, personalized weight control programme has not been a sudden thing but has evolved over a long period of time. It has become a way of life for you. You have not crash dieted or fasted and therefore your weight is very unlikely to pile back on as soon as your goals have all been attained. You have exercised and maintained or even increased your metabolic rate so that you can still eat reasonable, good-sized meals and not add body fat.

Once your goals have been reached and all your rewards earned, you can stop keeping a detailed diary. However, do not throw it away. Keep it to glance through occasionally (as you should glance through your photo album showing your changing shape) to remind you of the progress you have made. This should help motivate you to maintain your change. Your new low-fat, low-sugar, low-salt, high-fibre way of eating should be enjoyable enough to become a permanent way of life and be a tremendous help in preventing you from regaining weight.

We do strongly recommend that you continue to weigh yourself regularly. When your programme is fully finished, continue to weigh each day for a few months. If your weight increases by a few pounds (about 1 kg) from one day to the next, do nothing for a day or two to try to redress the balance; your weight could well drop back quite naturally. If, however, your weight stays at this higher level for four or five days, take the necessary measures to bring it back down. Eat slightly less and exercise a little more; aim to bring it back to normal within a week or two. After two or three months of keeping to your correct weight you should feel confident that you are really in control and you can now start to weigh yourself every other day rather than each day. Eventually it should be quite sufficient to weigh yourself once every week or two.

Although you will no longer be keeping a diary once your programme is completed, it is an excellent idea to retain certain interests like seeking out new recipes, experimenting with different foods, trying new sports, improving your exercise capability. These new pleasures should reinforce your committment to a healthier way of life.

Finally, now that you have achieved control over your weight, how has this changed you as a person? Your attitude to life should be far more positive and your self-esteem justifiably high. You should also find you have capabilities you never dreamed of. What you have learned is a sophisticated procedure for helping you solve difficult problems. You have learned to look hard and analyse a complex situation, devise a detailed strategy for solving it, and then carefully carry it out over a period of time, revising your plan where necessary to cope with unforeseen difficulties. These general problem-solving strategies can be used to help you through many of life's problems. By breaking a task down into small, manageable pieces, keeping reward levels high and taking an analytical approach you can achieve a great deal in all spheres of life. You will also understand yourself more, you will have a better idea of what motivates you. Your success with your weight control programme will make you healthy and fit enough to enjoy many different aspects of life.

Index